# Vent Hero: Advanced Transport Ventilator Management

Charles F. Swearingen

ISBN: 1530918243
ISBN-13:9781530918249

# DEDICATION

I have had continued family support throughout all of my endeavors. My mother, Jan Swearingen, and late father, Gene Swearingen, armed me with both an incredible work ethic and respect for integrity. Along the way, I developed a love for knowledge and respect for science which pair well with that integrity and work ethic.

My sister, Susan, is the eternal optimist and always has a smile on her face or laughter in her voice. I have learned so much from her by observing her through adversity and smiling her way through it.

I have incredible aunts who have always shown me love, and I credit them, along with my parents, with whatever kindness that I have developed. Aunt Susan, Carrie, Linda, and Rebecca, thank you for your continued love and support in all I have attempted.

I also have incredible cousins. Cindy, thank you for the long nights where I would cry to you about life's problems. You have always been there for me and I'll always love you for it. Jenny, you too have stayed up with me and shared advice. It means the world that you two have helped me through so much. I love you both. Katie, you are the sweetest lady I know. Thank you for showing me how to truly 'kill people with kindness.' Megan, I love how eccentric you are. I think you have a very unique eye for life. Tim , man do you set the bar high! You always have such a positive attitude and gratitude for life and your company is infectious. I love being around you. Thanks for always caring in the right ways and for the right reasons. You are truly one of a kind.

My grandmother, Marjorie Priester, is the epitome of a southern lady. She helped instill in me the persona of a southern gentleman and taught me that manners should always be practiced. I thank you for every ounce of the love you have given me. I love you so much.

And finally to my wife, who painstakingly edited this book , I thank you for your continued support in my endeavors. To have someone so devoted to those little things that feed my professional desires humbles me to what kind of woman is in my life. You are what drives me to begin and finish projects like and provide me with love and strength throughout.

Thank you for  your love and strength.

I love you.

# CONTENTS

# REVIEWER ACKNOWLEDGMENTS

Kevin King, RN, NRP, FP-C, CFRN
Flight Nurse, AirCare
University of Mississippi Health Care
Jackson, MS

Ken Walters, BS, NRP, CCEMT-P
Paramedic/ Field Training Officer
American Medical Response
Jackson, MS

Michael Boulding, NRP
Flight Paramedic, San Antonio Air Life
San Antonio, TX

Tony Harrison, NRP, FP-C
Flight Nurse and
Regional Clinical Compliance Manager
Air Methods
Somerset, KY

# 1
## BASIC VENTILATOR REVIEW

The core body of literature concerning air medical transport reports a reduced mortality when a flight paramedic and a flight nurse, together, transport sick and injured patients. A John Hopkins study in 2013 suggested that this mortality can be reduced to a magnitude of 15%. When they investigated why the reduced mortality occurs, they discovered that other than the pairing of the nurse and paramedic, their utilization of a mechanical ventilator significantly aided to the decreased mortality.

This seems like great news, if we, as a group, were proficient at using the mechanical ventilator. If you were to ask any co-worker or transport clinical personnel to describe basic functions of the mechanical ventilator or mechanical ventilation, chances are you're not going to get a very thorough answer. From years in this field I have discovered there is one singular skill that we in the air medical and transport communities are horrible at- the use of the mechanical ventilator.

So, we are not proficient at mechanical ventilation. Consider this: how much more mortality could possibly be reduce if we became proficient at this skill? I must commend and applaud you for your endeavor to better your knowledge and skill in mechanical ventilation because it is one of the defining elements in transport medicine that can truly save lives.

As with any skill, procedure, or competency, we must first have a solid knowledge base and understand the smaller moving parts of a bigger complex system. In the following pages of this chapter we will investigate these small cogs of mechanical ventilation and begin to explain how they tie into complex mechanical ventilation concepts.

## THE MINUTE VENTILATION CONCEPT

To overcome the learning curve of the mechanical ventilator, I would like to first employ the concept of minute ventilation. Minute ventilation is the amount of air we breathe in and out in a single minute. It inversely correlates with our end tidal carbon dioxide (EtCO2); if minute ventilation increases, then EtCO2 will decrease. Too often, I hear clinicians discussing adjusting the respiratory rate or tidal volume without mention of the minute ventilation. This makes as much sense as administering a fluid bolus and not checking the blood pressure afterwards.

The concept of minute ventilation is used by physicians, respiratory therapists, and savvy transport clinicians to guide their clinical decision making with respect to the mechanical ventilator. Simply defined, the minute ventilation (VE) is the respiratory rate (RR) multiplied by the tidal volume (Vt); or [VE = RR x Vt]. It can be monitored by the patient's pH or EtCO2. In critical care transport, we may not always have up to the minute ABG data, but we can always monitor EtCO2. In doing so, we can utilize end-tidal CO2 as a reliable estimate of the pH. For example, consider a patient with a RR of 15 bpm and a Vt of 450 cc. Their minute ventilation would be 6.75 L/min. If their EtCO2 was 62 mmHg, would this minute ventilation be sufficient? Absolutely not! So, to correct this high EtCO2, we need to increase the minute ventilation. To do that, we'll need to raise either the RR or the Vt.

Maintaining a minute ventilation to achieve an EtCO2 with the normal range of 35- 45 mmHg is imperative to the 'stickiness' of oxygen to the red blood cell (RBC). EtCO2 that is less than 35 mmHg makes the RBC incredibly "sticky" and once at the tissue beds, oxygen will not be able to break off of the RBCs and enter the tissues. If the EtCO2 is higher than 45 mmHg, then the RBC isn't very sticky at all and fails to collect enough oxygen molecules at the alveolar capillary membrane. If we maintain an end-tidal CO2 in our patients between 35-45 mmHg, then we can be assured that we are maximizing oxygen on loading onto the red blood cell and oxygen offload as the red blood cell passes through capillaries within tissues.

Throughout this text, the concept of mechanical ventilation will be discussed and put into practice by several practice sessions spread out throughout the book. It is a cornerstone in appropriately initiating and maintaining mechanical ventilation. It is imperative that each time a change in RR or Vt is made, one realization should develop in your mind: "I just changed minute ventilation."

## PRACTICE SESSION #1:

1. You notice someone in the airport breathing 14 breaths per minute. They are calmly inhaling and you assume they have a tidal volume of 500 cc. What is their expected minute ventilation?
2. You notice the patient on the ventilator with the following settings: RR 18, TV 450. What is their expected minute ventilation?
3. Your patient has an EtCO2 of 60, RR of 20 and a Vt of 450. Which of the following would correct the EtCO2?
   a. Lower minute ventilation
   b. Increase the RR to 24
   c. Reduce the Vt to 400
   d. Increase the EtCO2

## VOLUME CONTROL VERSUS PRESSURE CONTROL

Now we will discuss volume ventilation versus pressure ventilation. This typically is the first selection you will make when applying a mechanical ventilator to your patient. A transport ventilator will deliver air into a patient's chest until either a certain volume is reached or a certain pressure is reached. The clinician decides which "stopping point" best suits the patient.

This first decision has been traditionally based on age. Pediatrics receive pressure and adults receive volume. Sound familiar? Clinicians have historically used pressure in children as a protective measure to prevent barotrauma. Conversely, adults have been provided volume ventilation because it is less likely to cause barotrauma on most patients even with mild- moderately diseased lungs. Additionally, it is easier to control minute ventilation while in volume ventilation. However, the volume versus pressure decision is actually best made by considering the condition of the patient's lung. I will soon offer a universal approach to applying and adjusting the mechanical ventilator which takes into account the patient's minute ventilation status and their lung condition, or compliance.

Volume Control Ventilation

Volume ventilation is a particular breath type, or ventilation, that is characterized by advancing air into the lungs until a certain volume is reached and then the ventilator stops its inspiratory cycle and allows for exhalation. With this breath type, you can always guarantee a specific minute ventilation, allowing you to drive the patient's end-tidal $CO_2$ (or pH) towards a direction that maximizes oxygen on load and offload relative to the red blood cell. It is therefore incredibly important that we work hard on 99% of the patients to obtain $EtCO_2$ readings within normal ranges.

Patients who benefit from volume ventilation (also called volume control ventilation) include those that have relatively healthy lungs as well as the adult population in general. It is desirable because we can control minute ventilation better than we can in pressure control, and therefore can better control the pH. However, it does not come without drawbacks. Volume control ventilation is a generally a poor mode with respect to younger pediatric patients in general (infants and toddlers) as well as patients with injured or diseased lungs, such as adult respiratory distress syndrome (ARDS) and acute lung injury (ALI). Older pediatric patients (school age and older) can accept volume control ventilation better than infants and toddlers due to their more developed pulmonary system. The stigma of not using volume control in infants and toddlers is the danger of forcing in the a large volume of air and causing barotrauma from exceeding > 30 cmH2O of plateau pressure (which we'll discuss later). As a clinician, if you establish volume control ventilation in an infant, be sure to monitor the plateau pressures.

The most prominent benefit of volume control ventilation is the ability to completely control the minute ventilation. As previously mentioned, we can drive our patient's physiology (control EtCO2, and thus pH) by changing the minute ventilation. The concept of minute ventilation has been used by physicians, respiratory therapists, and savvy transport clinicians to guide their clinical decision making with respect to the mechanical ventilator. In critical care transport, we may not always have ABG data, but we can always monitor EtCO2, so we utilize end-tidal CO2 as a reliable estimate of the pH.

### When to Select Volume Control:
1. Healthy (non- diseased) lungs
2. Any patient age range, but be careful to never exceed a plateau pressure of 30 cmH2O; especially in smaller pediatrics and infants.

Pressure Control Ventilation

Pressure control ventilation is characterized by the delivery of air into a lung until a certain pressure is reached, at which point the inspiratory cycle ceases and exhalation is allowed. This breath type is utilized often with pediatric patients and patients in whom have diseased lungs (ARDS or ALI). Pressure control is a fantastic breath type because it allows you to set a maximum pressure. Once this max pressure is set, then the ventilator will fill the lungs until that pressure, and then cease inspiration. The true benefit of pressure control is being able to prevent a dangerously high maximum pressures from ever happening.

A common pressure control setting for all patient types is 18-22 cm H2O. The popular way to describe pressure control is in the form of a fraction: provide "20 over 5" as a starting point, which is 20 cmH2O of pressure control and cmH2O of PEEP. Another example would be "16 over 4", which is a common neonate setting where you are providing pressure control of 16 and a PEEP of 4.

### When to Select Pressure Control:
1. Diseased lungs
2. Smaller pediatric patients (infants and toddlers)

Too often, transport clinicians often shy away from of pressure control, but typically it is because it is not well understood. Most ventilator textbooks and literature will mention that in volume control, the pressure is variable; and that while in pressure control, volume is variable. This explanation seems vague and incomplete. To understand pressure control, let's first put it in practical terms.

Consider, for example, applying a mechanical ventilator to an adult patient and adjusting the settings to the following: 12 breaths per minute and a tidal volume of 500 cc. Now when you multiply 12 and 500 ccs, you get 6000 ccs, which is 6 liters. So on volume control ventilation, you can set a tidal volume of 500cc, you can set that respiratory rate or 12 and the patient is set to receive a minute ventilation of 6 liters.

You can accomplish the same goal of targeting a minute ventilation while in pressure control, but you need to take an additional step. In pressure control, you would set the pressure control setting, and then watch a variable that the ventilator measures called, exhaled tidal volume (Vte). To do this, you would set the PC setting to 20, and then monitor Vte to see how much tidal volume the patient is receiving. The Vte represents the patient's REAL tidal volume. What comes out of the patient is the best representation of what actually went into the patient. In volume control, we set the Vt in hopes they receive this volume, and the Vte informs us whether we are hitting our mark or not. In pressure control, we set the PC (20 cmH2O is a good starting point), check Vte to see how much tidal volume we actually are moving with each breath, and then we adjust the PC setting up or down to target our desired Vt.

---

**<u>VENT HERO SECRET #1</u>: You can still aim for a specific minute volume in PRESSURE CONTROL ventilation.**

---

Another way to explain this is to describe how a marksman hits a target at a shooting range. The marksman looks down range at his target. He then will expand his vision and determine how strong the wind is because this will affect the flight path of the bullet. If the wind is strong and he aims directly at the target, the wind will push the bullet away from the target and he will have to score a "miss." The marksman will have to overcome the wind effect. If the wind is moving from left to right, then he would need to aim left of the target to hit it. This is exactly what we do when we set up volume control or pressure control. We target a Vt based on their ideal body weight (soon to be discussed), or IBW. We will aim for this target as we set the ventilator to deliver this volume. Once the pressure control or volume control settings are applied, then we simply monitor the Vte to see if we are on target. If we are off target, just like the marksman and the wind, we will need to adjust PC (if using pressure control) or the Vt (if in volume control) to push our Vte closer to our targeted Vt.

So if you set a pressure control of 20 cmH2O on a patient and you allow a few breaths go by, you need to look at the monitored data on the ventilator for the variable Vte. Should you be targeting a Vte of 450 cc and your Vte is reported at 650 cc, then you would need to adjust the PC setting to a lower value. In general, small adjustments are a good idea because you gain a familiarity with the magnitude of the change based on your adjustment. In this case, if you reduce your PC setting to 18 cmH2O and the Vte changes to 550 cc, then you are aware that a 2 cmH20 change should be close to equaling a change in

Vte of about 100 cc. These ratios will change from patient to patient, so it is not necessary to memorize this PC to Vte ratio. Since we are not yet at our target, let's make another change of 2 cmH2O. We adjust the PC setting from 18 cmH2O to 16 cmH2O and after a few breaths we note a Vte of 465 cc. This isn't perfect, but it never will be. This would be a successful adjustment since we are now at our target Vt as proven by the Vte. So, you can't specifically dial in a tidal volume while in pressure control, but you can adjust the pressure control setting up or down to get drive your Vte to the desired level.

The first question you need to answer when applying a mechanical ventilator is simply do we need to apply pressure control or do they need volume control? Traditionally, patients with damaged lungs (ARDS or acute lung injury) or pediatric patients receive pressure control. Volume control has been traditionally utilized in the adult and larger pediatric populations, as well as with patients with relatively healthy lungs. While this is just a general guideline, it does not necessarily matter which breath type is chosen over the other, initially, as long as in volume control you never deliver a breath that measures over 30 cm H2O of plateau pressure. Doing so can cause barotrauma and damage the lungs. In the past, pressure control has been utilized with children because it is easier to protect the patient from an inexperienced clinician manipulating mechanical ventilation. However, it is safe to apply volume ventilation on a 1 month old pediatric, if you are watching their pressures and ensuring they do not exceed 30 cmH2O of plateau pressure.

### General Initial Pressure vs. Volume Guidelines:
1. Infants: Pressure control
2. Pediatrics & Adults: Volume control

As clinicians, we need to be fluid in our decision making. If we apply a guideline such as "infants should be initially placed on pressure control ventilation", but we determine they need to be on volume control (perhaps to better control their minute ventilation) then we need to be prepared to make those changes. This concept of fluidity in clinical decision making will apply to all future sections of this text. We should always be assessing our patients and making clinical decisions to better their outcomes. If you simply set the default settings on your transport ventilator and fail to assess and reassess your patient then you are not practicing appropriate medicine.

## PRACTICE SESSION #2:

1. You are transporting an 11 month old patient with pneumonia. You intubate the patient and will now apply the mechanical ventilator. Which of the following are appropriate initial settings? Circle one: Volume or Pressure.
2. Your patient is a middle-aged adult who presents with an AMI and is being transferred to a cath lab. The sending facility intubated your patient just prior to your arrival and is currently bagging with a BVM. Which of the following are appropriate initial settings? Circle one: Volume or Pressure.
3. An adult patient has the following ventilator findings: PC 17 cmH2O and Vte 300cc. You calculate tidal volume to be 450cc. How will you adjust the ventilator to achieve the target Vt of 450cc?

## COMMON MODES OF VENTILATION

Modes dictate what happens when the patient tries to initiate a breath. If the patient never attempts to ventilate or to take a breath on their own, then the mode itself does not matter. The ventilator will default to the preset rate and either the preset tidal volume (if you set volume control ventilation) or the preset pressure control (if you set the ventilator to pressure control ventilation). Therefore, if a patient is appropriately sedated and/or paralyzed, the mode will not matter because they will be too medicated to initiate a breath. Yes– it is that simple.

There are three basic modes that we will first discuss and practice using: CMV, A/C, and SIMV. In a much later chapter and after we have sufficiently covered these three basic modes, an advanced mode,

PRVC, will be discussed and practiced. As with any other skill, we must learn the basics before proceeding to the advanced level.

---

**Vent Hero Rule #2**: If your patient is chemically paralyzed, or adequately sedated, then the ventilator mode you apply doesn't matter. Mode decides what the ventilator will do if they are awake to take a breath and there is no need to attempt vent weaning in transport medicine.

---

Controlled Mandatory Ventilation (CMV)

Of the three most common types of transport ventilator modes (the first and the simplest) is controlled mandatory ventilation or CMV. CMV is characterized by defining a preset tidal volume or pressure control, and a preset respiratory rate. It has no bearing on breath attempts that patient may make. The patient will receive a set tidal volume or a set pressure at the specific rate that is dialed into the ventilator. This is not a very advanced mode of ventilation because the machine fails to respond to the patient initiating his own breath(s). It **IS** used, commonly, in the neonate sector of transport medicine.

Consider the patient who is preset to receive 20 breaths per minute (bpm) and 500 cc per breath. At these settings, patient will receive one 500 cc tidal volume every 3 seconds, and obviously is in volume control. The ventilator set to CMV will deliver one 500 cc breath every 3 seconds. The ventilator will not change this pattern and is uninfluenced by any patient breath attempts. This type of mechanical ventilation is completely okay if the patient is paralyzed or for any reason will not take a breath (apneic). Any condition in which the patient will not be able to take a spontaneous breath, then controlled mandatory ventilation is suitable. However, if the patient has any ability to take a breath, then the patient is at risk for breath stacking, also known as auto-peep.

Consider the aforementioned scenario: the patient is receiving 20 breaths per minute and 500 ccs. What happens when the patient takes a breath in between the machine-delivered ventilations? During this time the patient is allowed to take a breath on their own without any effect on the ventilator itself. But what happens if the patient tries to take a breath, brings in their full tidal volume, say 450 cc, at the exact moment that the mechanical ventilator is about to deliver its breath? When the patient has all of their tidal volume in their chest (450 cc) and the machine delivers a breath right on top of it, it is referred to as breath stacking. Breath stacking is very dangerous because it can damage lung tissue, an injury known as barotrauma. This is the danger in controlled mandatory ventilation: if you fail to adequately sedate or paralyze your patient and they try to take a breath the moment that the mechanical ventilator is about to deliver a breath, then they risk stacking breaths and causing damage to the lung tissue by barotrauma.

Assist Control Ventilation (A/C)

Somewhere along the way somebody figured out that if we designed a mechanical ventilator that can deliver a breath, but sense when the patient takes a breath, then we might be able to devise a mode that would protect a patient from this breath stacking phenomenon. This is called assist control mode ventilation, or A/C.. In A/C mode, you choose a preset rate and either tidal volume or pressure, just like in other modes, only this mode will monitor for patient breathing attempts. If the patient takes a breath, the machine automatically recognizes it and delivers a full preset tidal volume or pressure control breath at the very beginning of the patient's inspiration. What this means is, as soon as the patient begins to take a breath, the ventilator recognizes it and delivers the pre-set tidal volume or pressure. If the patient is completely paralyzed or very well sedated, then this mode will behave just like a controlled mandatory ventilation and deliver its present tidal volume or pressure at the prescribed and dialed-in rate. Therefore, the biggest benefit of A/C ventilation is that the ventilator assists the patient each time they begin to initiate a breath, thereby preventing the potential for breath stacking and reducing the potential for barotrauma.

The danger of this mode is high and uncontrolled minute ventilation. Imagine a patient who is not well sedated and who is breathing faster than the preset rate. If this occurs, then the patient is increasing the minute ventilation, which can quickly lower the patient's $CO_2$ and elevate their pH. If the patient remains under-sedated, the patient will continue to breathe faster, thereby moving more air within a minute than the clinician originally set on the ventilator. For instance, if we set on the ventilator 20 breaths per minute and 500 ccs per breath, then over the course of one minute, the patient will move 10 liters {20 x 500cc = 10,000 cc = 10L). So if this is the case and your patient breathes faster than 20 times a minute, then that 10L/min minute ventilation will elevate even further. If your patient was breathing 26/min, then 26 times per minute the A/C mode would fill the patient's lungs with 500 cc. Therefore, the minute ventilation would be 13 L/min instead of 10 L/min, which would drive down the EtCO2 and drive up the pH (causing acidosis).

Synchronized Intermittent Mandatory Ventilation (SIMV)

Later, a clever scientist figured they needed to upgrade the abilities of the ventilator even further. Assist control mode prevents breath stacking, however allows the patient to hyperventilate over the pre-set respiratory rate, thereby increasing the minute ventilation to potentially dangerous levels. This led to the invention of SIMV mode.

The SIMV mode is initiated similar to other modes. You choose a preset volume (or pressure if choosing pressure control ventilation) to be delivered at a preset rate. Similar to all the other modes, this mode is *specific* to what happens when the patient takes a breath. If the patient is adequately sedated or paralyzed, then the patient will never take a breath and therefore will not trigger the characteristics of the SIMV mode.

The SIMV mode works by ensuring the pre-set rate is delivered without breath stacking and prevents excessive minute ventilation. This is accomplished by the microprocessor inside and the algorithms programmed into the ventilator. It prevents excessive minute ventilation by occasionally allowing the patient to take in a breath completely under their own power. If you set the RR of 12, then the ventilator will identify how many breaths the patient is taking and how many breaths are machine driven. It will synchronize the patient's efforts and fill in any needed machine breaths to ensure the pre-set respiratory rate is met. If the patient is apneic, then the SIMV mode will deliver 12 breaths. If the patient is taking 6 breaths per minute then the vent will deliver only 6 breaths per minute. If the patient is breathing over 12 breaths per minute, the ventilator will try to figure out the best combination of patient-triggered breaths to machine breaths.

To understand how SIMV works, you need to think of umbrellas. This mode will conceptually have "umbrellas", like windows of opportunity, as time progresses. A patient who attempts a breath in SIMV mode has two outcomes: 1) the patient receives a full preset Vt or PC ventilation, or 2) the patient is allowed to take as large a breath as they can muster under their own power. The outcome is determined by a point in time when the patient attempts their breath. If the patient attempts a ventilation under the "umbrella", they receive a full preset tidal volume or pressure control breath just like in A/C mode. If the patient breathes outside the "umbrella", then the patient receives whatever they can bring down on their own power.

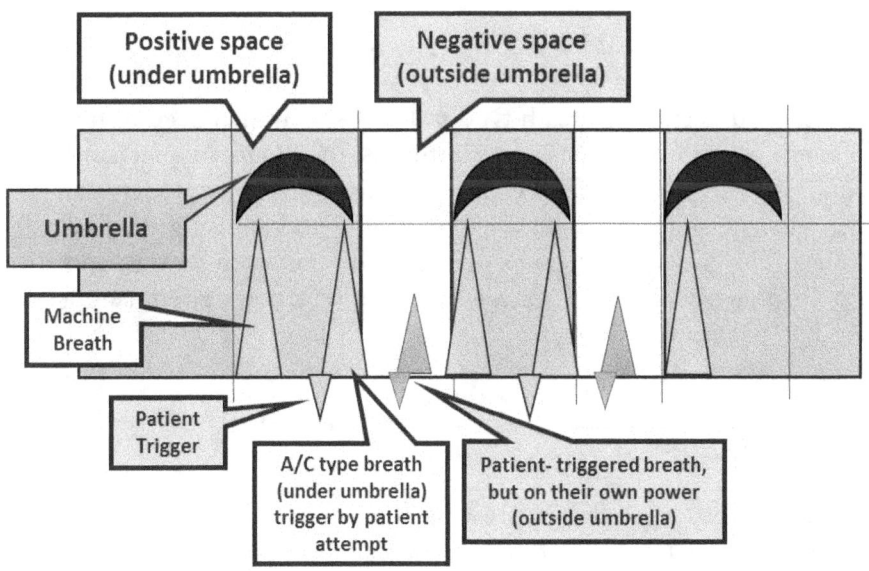

You see, the SIMV mode has specific programmed intervals that come into play when the patient takes a breath on their own. One type of interval correlates with a full tidal volume breath. We've described these intervals as "umbrellas". Another type of interval in the programming is a breath that is attempted by the patient where they are allowed to inspire on their own power, which is the interval we describe as "outside the umbrella". We cannot control these intervals or programming with transport ventilators, however, we can learn how to best operate them. Also, the programming and the microprocessor in the ventilator itself decides the dimensions of these intervals. You just need to remember that with SIMV some patient attempts are delivered as a full pre-set breath (just like an A/C breath) and other patient attempts are allowed, but the patient has to inspire completely under their own power.

One concept that we will mention now and further discuss in a later section is pressure support (PS). Pressure support is a setting that can be applied in either volume control ventilation or pressure control ventilation, but can only be applied in the SIMV mode. Since the SIMV mode allows the patient to take breaths on their own power (and other modes do not allow for this) we as clinicians can decide to apply a little 'turbo boost' upon their efforts or allow them power their own breath.

## VENTILATOR SETTINGS

After you decide on breath type and mode, you then need to input the settings into the ventilator. If this is the point in mechanical ventilation that you begin to become anxious, you are not alone. Many flight clinicians are uncertain when choosing and applying ventilator settings. This section will cover the basics of ventilator settings and a later chapter will dive into a more advanced selection of vent settings based on patient condition.

Respiratory Rate

Respiratory rate (RR) represents the default rate in which the ventilator will deliver a breath to a patient. Typically, the rate is either set to a value within the normal respiratory range for the patient's age, or is set outside the range to help achieve a desired minute ventilation. Remember, minute ventilation is the respiratory rate multiplied by the tidal volume [VE = RR x Vt]. Additionally, anytime that the RR is adjusted on the mechanical ventilator an immediate correlation should be made with minute ventilation.

The normal respiratory rate for an adult is 12-20 breaths/min, a pediatric is 20-30/min, and an infant is 30-40/min. Patients can be set on the ventilator within these ranges, or can be set outside these ranges within reason. A respiratory rate for an adult could be set lower than 12, as long as there is a deliberate and cautious reason to do so. For instance, you could set an adult patient to receive 8 breaths/min if the EtCO2 was slightly low at 32 mmHg. Conversely, it is reasonable to set a RR to 26 breaths/min in an adult patient if their EtCO2 was high. I must caution you, however, that in each age range you reach a respiratory rate so high you can cause breath stacking. This breath stacking is caused by breathing so fast that exhalation is interrupted before the next inhalation. **Anytime there is incomplete exhalation there will be breath stacking.** As a rule of thumb: the closer you get to 10 above the highest normal value for an age range, breath stacking will most likely occur. Being able to identify breath stacking, also called AutoPEEP, is an upcoming Vent Hero © secret in a later chapter.

Tidal Volume

The tidal volume (Vt) is set when delivering breaths while using volume control ventilation and represents the volume in a single breath. Normal tidal volume is derived from a simple calculation involving the patient's ideal body weight (IBW) and the widely accepted range for appropriate tidal volume (5-8 cc/kg). Just like RR, anytime you reach over to adjust the Vt on the mechanical ventilator, you are effectively changing the minute ventilation. Additionally, you should always reference the peak pressures after each increase in Vt to insure the extra volume is not causing dangerously high pressures. Shortly, we will discuss normal pressure ranges and how to use them clinically.

As mentioned in the previous paragraph, there is a calculation to determine a patient's tidal volume based on their ideal body weight (IBW). To correctly obtain the patient's Vt, we'll need to make two separate and simple calculations. The first is the IBW. The IBW formula is [IBW in Kg = 2.3 x (height in inches - 60 inches) + (50 for males; 45.5 for females). This is an easy calculation. The "height in inches - 60 inches" term simply means to take the patient's height and take 5 feet (or 60 inches) away. The remaining number of inches gets multiplied by 2.3. The result is then added to 50 if the patient is a male or 45.5 if the patient is female. This formula is called the Devine formula for IBW calculation and is widely accepted in medical literature. Additionally, this becomes very easy after practicing even just a few times.

Once you have the patient's IBW, you simply choose a value within the accepted Vt range. Remember, normal Vt is 5-8 cc/kg. I personally like the middle numbers, 6 and 7, because, well, they are in the middle. Choose one right for your patient and multiply it by their IBW. The result yields the ideal tidal volume (ITV) for that patient. Please note: ideal tidal volume is a "Charlie Swearingen" term and not a largely accepted term. The rest of the terms described will be consistent with the nomenclature of respiratory therapy and critical care medicine.

## PRACTICE SESSION #3:

1. Your female patient is 5'9". What is her IBW?
2. Your male patient is 6'3" and weighs 350 pounds. What is his IBW?
3. What is the ideal tidal volume for a 6'1" female who weighs 132 lbs?

Pressure Control

The pressure control (PC) is set when delivering breaths while using pressure control ventilation and represents the maximum inspiratory pressure in a single breath. This is a unique setting in that the standard and normal range is good for all ages. The universally accepted normal range is 18-22 cmH2O. As mentioned earlier in this chapter, the PC setting involves pushing air into a patient's chest until a particular pressure is reached. At this point, inspiration is halted and expiration is allowed to begin. By setting a specific pressure to end inspiration, we can only be hopeful that the right amount of volume enters the patient's lungs.

We can, however, gauge to see how much air enters our patient's lungs with each breath- as we have already discussed. By observing the Vte, also called the exhaled tidal volume, while in pressure control ventilation, we can get an idea on how much air is actually entering the lungs. We can use the Vte as a surrogate tidal volume. This is the main premise to the argument that you can still control minute ventilation while in pressure control ventilation. Since the pressure control setting prevents damaging delicate lung tissue by limiting the maximum pressure during an inspiration, you can keep a set pressure and target a minute ventilation using the Vte and RR. So, just like RR and Vt, PC effects the minute ventilation.

I:E Ratio

It takes humans about one second to take in a full breath and two seconds to fully exhale. During inspiration, our diaphragm is stimulated to contract and the umbrella-shaped muscle swiftly flattens. This increases the volume in the chest causing a reduction in pressure within the lung. The higher outside pressure of the atmosphere rushes into the lungs. Once full, the nervous signal telling the diaphragm to remain contracted is ceased, and it is allowed to relax. As the diaphragm relaxes, the volume in the chest is slowly reduced causing increased intrathroacic pressure. The built up higher pressure in the chest then pushes its way out of the lung, typically slower than it took to inhale. When we set the I:E ratio, we attempt to mirror this physiology.

Normally, I:E will be appropriate at 1:2, meaning one full respiratory cycle (the time for one inspiration and one exhalation) is one part inhalation and two parts exhalation. The time it takes for inhalation is called the I- time, and conversely, the time it takes to exhale is the E-time. An I:E of 1:2 is appropriate in any patient who can mimic the normal exhalation physiology. Most adult patients with healthy lungs will fall into this category. However, this will not apply to some patients with diseased lungs, airways, or small pediatric patients who do not yet have a well-developed respiratory system. These patients cannot mimic normal exhalation physiology, and so need to be provided more time to exhale. In patients with any bronchospasm (asthma, COPD) or in smaller pediatrics, longer E-times should be administered. We accomplish this by adjusting the I time setting higher or lower to achieve an I:E ratio of 1:4, 1:5, or 1:6. The monitored data panel will be the source where this ratio will be displayed.

Most transport ventilators, however, do not allow you to directly change the I:E ratio and require you change the I-time setting. For respiratory therapists, the I-time may be important, but for transport clinicians I argue that the I:E ratio is much more valuable. The I time is just a means to get to an I:E ratio, meaning the I time is just a setting but choosing an appropriate I:E ratio based on your patient's condition is much more therapeutic. Remember the marksman analogy. The I-time is our 'aim' and the I:E ratio is our actual 'bullseye'. If your patient is a pediatric or has a disease characterized by bronchospasm, you'll need to adjust your I time (aim) to achieve a I:E ratio of 1:4 to 1:6 (the bullseye).

It should be mentioned that most transport ventilators force you to change the I:E ratio by selecting and adjusting the I-time. What I usually advised is to select the I-time button, cover the number up with your thumb, turn the adjustment knob and watch the I:E ratio change on the display panel. By utilizing this method of covering the actual I-time value you can focus your eyes and attention on the I:E ratio. As it changes, it allows you to stop on the specific setting you want to target. Luckily, when you select the I-time button, most transport ventilators automatically display the I:E ratio on the display panel.

Transport ventilators will hold I-time constant when you adjust the respiratory rate. This means each time you change the respiratory rate (and I-time is held constant) you also change the I:E ratio. Therefore, you should always re-check your I:E ratio <u>after each change in RR</u> to ensure your I:E ratio is still set to the setting you desire for the patient.

<u>**Vent Hero Rule #3**</u>: **With a transport ventilator, every time you re-adjust respiratory rate, then re-adjust the I:E ratio.**

Positive End Expiratory Pressure (PEEP)

The positive end expiratory pressure, or PEEP, essentially is the air pressure that's left in the lungs after exhalation, or the residual pressure after most of the air has been exhaled. You can imagine PEEP as an invisible pressure-driven scaffolding that holds open alveoli. That's all it really does. Alveoli have a tendency to collapse, and infected or inflamed alveoli will have a difficult time reopening in addition to causing further damage with the re- opening process itself. Therefore, holding open alveoli is in the patient's best clinical interest.

While the gas laws of flight physiology are mostly outside the scope of this text, there is one that remains pertinent: Fick's Law, because it describes how PEEP works. Fick's Law describes improved gaseous diffusion in a membrane with more surface area as well as with a thinner membrane. By increasing the PEEP in your patients, you are essentially increasing the surface area of the alveoli (because you're making them bigger) and thinning out the alveolar capillary membrane (oxygen crosses a thinner membrane faster than a thicker membrane). This is much like a balloon. By inflating a balloon, you increase the size (surface area) and reduce its thickness (thin the membrane). These mechanisms allow for greater oxygen into the blood stream, and the more blood available to the tissues. Therefore, a thin alveolar-capillary membrane that increased PEEP causes greater oxygen diffusion, thus improving pulse oximetry and increasing PaO2.

It should be mentioned that as you increase PEEP beyond the highest normal value of 5 cmH2O, we start applying a massive dose of positive pressure to the alveoli and the alveolar-capillary membrane. This compression on the alveolar- capillary membrane stunts blood flow through the alveolar capillary. When you multiply this across both lungs, you get a significant reduction in cardiac output. A reduction in cardiac output can result in a drop in blood pressure. Typically, you will not get significant drops in blood pressure until you are applying 7-8 cmH2O of PEEP.

---

**Vent Hero Rule #4**: **If PEEP earns you improved oxygenation but drops BP, do not remove PEEP! Instead support BP with fluids, blood and/or pressors.**

---

In an upcoming section, we will revisit this concept of applying PEEP and then fluid to support any reductions in blood pressure due to the added PEEP.

A reasonable starting point for PEEP is between the ranges observed as normal: 3-5 cmH2O. As a critical care transport clinician, chances are your patients will be much sicker than non-critical care patients. For this reason, consider beginning at the higher side of the normal range. By starting at 4-5 cmH2O, you are beginning at the higher side of normal and giving a solid effort to keep the patient oxygenated. Later we will talk about a procedure to wean the patient from high amounts of supplemental oxygen, but for initial settings it is important to make sure your patient is well oxygenated.

### Fraction of Inspired Oxygen (FiO2)

FiO2 represents the percentage of air that is oxygen that goes into a mechanically ventilated patient. The range can be from 0.21 to 1.0 because room air is 21% oxygen while max oxygen is 100% FiO2. The fraction of inspired oxygen basically describes an increasing number of oxygen molecules into the patient's respiratory system. More oxygen molecules into the respiratory system means more oxygen at the alveolar capillary membrane and thus greater oxygen diffusion. We can increase the patient's oxygen saturation by increasing the FiO2.

It is wise to begin almost all of your patients for whom <u>you initiate</u>

mechanical ventilation with 1.0 FiO2. The danger with starting a lower FiO2 is hypoxia, which increases mortality (especially in trauma patients). If you start low and have to titrate up to get a pulse oximetry reading above 95%, you could be wasting valuable, life-saving time. Conversely, if you go straight to 1.0 then you can achieve appropriate oxygen saturations earlier and avoid further hypoxic complications. Once you achieve an acceptable oxygen saturation (> 95%) at 1.0 FiO2, then you can begin titrating down the FiO2 (we will discuss this in a later chapter).

Pressure Support (PS)

When you decide to assist the patient with a "turbo boost" while in SIMV and on their self- driven effort, you can apply pressure support (normal starting point is 10 cmH2O of PS). Therefore, each time the patient is allowed to take a breath on their own (in SIMV only), you are instructing the ventilator to pressurize the airway which helps push in the breath they are working to pull into their lungs. Transport ventilators can only apply PS in SIMV because this is the only mode that allows the patient to inhale on their own power. It provides an opportunity for the clinician to apply a 'turbo boost' or to let them breathe completely on their own power. The advanced mode PRVC will be discussed later and is available on only a few transport ventilator models. The PRVC mode can also apply PS because it allows the patient to occasionally inhale completely on their own power- but again, it will be discussed later.

<u>Vent Hero Rule #5</u>: **Pressure support can only be applied in SIMV mode because it is the only ventilator mode where the patient has the ability to take a breath on their own power.**

**PRACTICE SESSION #4:**

1. What I:E ratio would you apply to a patient with a "shark fin" morphology on their EtCO2 waveform?

2. Your patient is on pressure control ventilation and the set PC is 19. Their Vte is 450 cc and their EtCO2 is 49 mmHg. What change can you make to drive this EtCO2 closer to the normal range?
3. What two settings can be changed to correct EtCO2?
4. What two settings can be changed to correct oxygenation problems?

## IMPORTANT PRESSURES

You should become familiar with two particular pressures on the mechanical ventilator: peak inspiratory pressure (PIP) and the plateau pressure (Pplat). These are two of the most important pressures when using mechanical ventilation. These pressures will assist the clinician identify different conditions the patient is experiencing as well as to identify the efficacy of volume ventilation. Additionally, mean airway pressure will also be discussed.

Peak Inspiratory Pressure (PIP)

The peak inspiratory pressure is the highest pressure the lungs experience during an inhalation, whether it be a spontaneous breath or machine driven. Like most pressures measured from the ventilator, PIP is measured in centimeters of water (cmH2O). Normal PIP for all age ranges is below 35 cmH2O. PIPs can be high in any condition that blocks the flow of gas into the lungs (secretions, bronchospasm, kinked endotracheal tubing), patient coughing (awake patients), and tension pneumothorax. The PIP can act as a whistleblower and alert us to potentially high pressures that could damage the lungs. A high PIP does not indicate lung damage or barotrauma, but it suggests that it could be happening.

Plateau Pressure

The plateau pressure is a direct reflection of the pressures the alveoli are experiencing and this pressure is greater than 30 cmH2O, lung tissue damage (barotrauma) is occurring. When high pressure alarms sound, you'll first rule out common causes of high PIP. Then, you will perform a maneuver on the ventilator which will provide you with the plateau pressure, information specific to the condition of the alveoli. The PIP simply *suggests* lung damage may be occurring, but the plateau pressure is <u>direct evidence</u> that lung damage is occurring.

---

**<u>Vent Hero Rule #6</u>: High PIP and normal pPlat = a resistance problem; high PIP and high pPlat = a compliance problem.**

---

Mean Airway Pressure (MAP)

The mean airway pressure is the average pressure exerted on the airway and lungs from the beginning of inspiration until the beginning of the next inspiration. It is one of the largest factors contributing to oxygenation. During inspiration, pressures in the lung increase, which increase the size of alveoli (increase their surface area) and thin the alveolar walls (increasing the rate of diffusion for gas exchange). During exhalation, the pressure that remains (positive end expiratory pressure, or PEEP) maintain a certain alveolar surface area and keep a somewhat thin alveolar membrane. Therefore, the mean pressure between the inspiratory and expiratory pressures dictate how long the alveoli are inflated and thinned, which speaks to oxygenation.

On the transport ventilator, we are limited in what we can achieve with respect to changing I times and E times. If you want to increase the I time, then you will change the I:E ratio. Increasing the I time shrinks your E time. Therefore, if you have an asthma patient and you want to increase their I time to improve oxygenation, that might work but it also could minimize the E time and cause air-trapping (also called autoPEEP). In transport ventilators, it is still a better idea to use PEEP and FiO2 to improve oxygenation, but I would remiss if I didn't mention the effect of I time.

## PRACTICE SESSION #5:

1. Explain the importance of peak inspiratory pressure.
2. Explain the importance of plateau pressure.
3. Why is mean airway pressure important in the inspiratory phase of ventilation?

## MISCELLANEOUS CONCEPTS

There are several settings that most transport ventilators will not allow you adjust. Remember, a transport ventilator has limited functionality compared to its hospital or ICU counterparts. This becomes confusing when you read other texts on mechanical ventilation where it mentions principles and settings that are not available on a transport ventilator. This section will provide a discussion on some of these principles and settings to provide a full and accurate review of the mechanical ventilator and arm you with the power to differentiate pertinent transport ventilator principles and settings.

Triggering and Sensitivity

Triggering is the determining factor that causes inspiration to begin. Ventilators may be triggered to deliver a breath based on time, pressure or flow. On a transport ventilator, the primary triggering variable is time, which can be recognized on the ventilator as respiratory rate. The secondary triggering variable is pressure. Yes, mechanical ventilators have secondary protocols for triggering, but we have no control over it and thus do not have to worry much about it. We set our initial settings and make changes according to SpO2 and EtCO2.

We can toggle the pressure trigger by changing the sensitivity setting. Sensitivity is the setting on the ventilator that represents the amount of inspiratory effort required by the patient's spontaneous effort to initiate a mechanically ventilated breath. Common settings for sensitivity are -1 to -2 cmH2O, meaning that the patient has to create a negative pressure breath to the magnitude of -1 to -2 cmH2O for the ventilator to register a spontaneous patient attempt. At that point, the ventilator would deliver a machine breath at the pre-set tidal volume (in in volume control ventilation) or pressure control (if in pressure control ventilation).

Modern ventilators utilize a flow-based mechanism where a small amount of gas is constantly flowing around the vent circuit, even during the pause from one exhalation to the next inhalation. When the patient takes a spontaneous breath, this flow is disrupted. The benefit of flow over pressure is that flow requires much less patient effort to trigger the breath which reduces the time from patient effort to the ventilator actually delivering the breath. However, most transport ventilators do not have this functionality.


Limiting

The limit is the setting that restricts the volume, pressure or time air is delivered to the patient during the inspiratory phase. On transport ventilator, we do not have a limiting setting control button. However, we indirectly set this when we choose volume control ventilation or pressure control ventilation. When we choose volume control ventilation we essentially are choosing out preset tidal volume as our limit. Once that volume has been reached, the ventilator will stop inputting air into the chest. With pressure control ventilation, the ventilator will cease inputting gas into the patient's lungs once the pressure control setting is reached. Again, on the transport ventilator you will not have to set the limit directly, but rather it will indirectly be selected when you choose pressure control or volume control. It is important I mention limit in this section for a full presentation of mechanical ventilation.


Cycling

Mechanical ventilator breaths can be divided into two distinctly different phases: inhalation and exhalation. As inhalation is coming to an end, gas flow into the lungs ceases, and the breath then enters the exhalation phase of the mechanically ventilated breath. The point where inspiration transitions into exhalation is referred to as the cycling point.

While this seems like an easy concept to understand, medical literature has offered multiple verbose nomenclature of it which complicates understanding. Cycling has also been termed "expiratory trigger," "inspiratory termination criteria," and "inspiratory flow termination." No matter what the name of this concept is, just remember it is the variable that determines the end- point of inspiration.

A mechanical ventilator will cycle after a set value is reached relative to a certain variable. For instance, if you set your ventilator on pressure control ventilation with a pressure control of 20 cmH2O, then what you've basically just done was to instruct the ventilator to cycle once a pressure of 20 cmH2O is reached. In this case, the variable is pressure and the set value is 20 cmH2O. If you were to apply volume control ventilation to a patient and you chose a tidal volume of 475 cc, then you are instructing the ventilator to cycle once 475 cc of gas is delivered to the patient.

## PRACTICE SESSION #6:

1. Explain what happens when sensitivity is set too low on the mechanical ventilator.
2. Describe how a mechanically ventilated breath progresses from inspiration to exhalation.
3. How is the inspiratory phase of a mechanically initiated breath halted?

Flow

Flow is like a nickname. This concept's formal name is peak inspiratory flow rate and it describes the speed at which the mechanical breath is delivered to the patient. It is how fast or how slow the breath is delivered. Flow can only be set in volume control ventilation. In pressure control ventilation the flowrates can vary significantly based on the condition of the patient's lungs (sick lungs will slow flowrates down) as well as some settings we apply to the ventilator such as I-time. Normal initial flow rates range from 40-60 liters per minute (LPM), however, flow rates can be adjusted between 20-120 LPM.

Flow rates are adjusted dependent on patient conditions. In theory, you want to target a flow rate that matches what the patient experiences when they are awake and breathing on their own. For instance, a COPD or asthma patients have increased airway resistance and would need a lower flow to achieve more evenly distributed gas with each inhalation. Conversely, patients with compliance related conditions (ARDS, pneumonia, etc.) would benefit from lower tidal volumes and higher inspiratory flow rates.

With most transport ventilators, we cannot actively change the flow rate. The transport ventilator will apply standard inspiratory flow rates based on the age level of your patient based on your choice of adult, pediatric, or infant. It is important to know how a transport ventilator limits the transport ventilator clinician, therefore, it was important to mention the mechanics of peak inspiratory flow.

Rise Time

Rise time refers to the time required by the ventilator to achieve the preset pressure during a machine- delivered breath in pressure control ventilation, pressure support ventilation, and even in pressure regulated volume control (PRVC) ventilation. The rise time can be conceptualized as a means to adjust the rate at which the ventilator establishes a preset pressure and indirectly controls peak flow. Several investigators have suggested using rise time to adjust flow delivery to establish a more synchronous interaction between ventilator and patient. By establishing a peak flow that is synchronous with the patient's ventilatory pattern and underlying lung disease, work of breathing can be optimized. Patients with airway resistance conditions benefit from lower rise times and patient's with lung compliance conditions benefit from higher rise times. Ultimately, rise time is a way to adjust the inspiratory flow rate (indirectly) on a transport ventilator when you are using a pressure- driven ventilator mode.

Total Cycle Time, Inspiratory Time and Expiratory Time

The total cycle time (TCT) is the total time of the respiratory cycle, so it is the inspiratory time (TI) plus the expiratory time(TE)

$$[ \text{TCT} = \text{TI} + \text{TE}]$$

Total cycle time is determined by the set respiratory rate. For example, if the set respiratory rate is 12 breaths per minute and the patient is not breathing above this set rate, the total cycle time is 5 seconds; if the respiratory rate is 20 breaths per minute, the total cycle time is 3 seconds. If you set your TI (time for inspiration), or I- time, to 1.0 with a respiratory rate of 20 breaths/min, then your TE (time of expiration), or E-time, would be 2 seconds. Therefore, your I:E ratio is 1:2. In transport, you will not have to routinely calculate TCT, I- times, or E-times. What will be more important and valuable to you is the I:E ratio, and luckily, the ventilator will measure that for you.

### PRACTICE SESSION #7:

1. How can flow rates be adjusted in the transport ventilators?
2. What type of patients could benefit from lower rise times in the transport ventilators?
3. Your patient is breathing 12 times per minute. If you set your I-time at 1.0, what is your I:E ratio?

### MANEUVERS

We have already discussed how powerful the mechanical ventilator is and how it can truly augment our patients pathophysiology to resemble physiology. This allows patients to heal, which really means allowing sugar and oxygen to act as energy to repair cells so they can comeback online physiologically. The transport ventilator has some features that allows you to monitor two variables to ensure your settings on the ventilator are benefiting the patient. Most transport ventilators have a maneuvers button that allows you to pause the ventilation. Doing so at various phases of the respiratory cycle gives you some incredibly useful information.

Inspiratory Hold Maneuver

The inspiratory hold maneuver is executed during <u>volume control ventilation</u> where the ventilator is told to pause the transition from inspiration to exhalation. This maneuver is used to identify the plateau pressure. Most transport ventilators have a "Maneuvers" button that when depressed will pause the respiratory cycle. Basically, during this maneuver inspiration is prolonged allowing gases to equalize within the deepest depths of the lung. The insight this provides the clinician is whether or not the lung is healthy and floppy, or if it is diseased and rigid. This information is presented by the ventilator in the form of plateau pressure (Pplat).

The plateau pressure represents the equalizing pressure of the lung. As air is forced into a lung under volume control ventilation, the pressure rises quickly and peaks (which is recorded as the peak inspiratory pressure). With the inspiratory hold maneuver, the respiratory cycle is paused at this point of maximal inspiration and the pressures within the lung are allowed to equalize. When the pressure equalizes, it lowers slightly. Normal physiology dictates a plateau pressure of less than 30 cmH2O to remain healthy, thus any breath experienced above this threshold (30 cmH2O) can damage the lung tissue.

The information provided by the plateau pressure is integral in handling a true high pressure alarm. When a high pressure alarm sounds, it is usually signaled by a high PIP. This is a poorly sensitive indicator to actual lung damage. A high PIP does not necessarily indicate lung damage because it could be caused by all kinds of physical mechanisms that do not involve diseased lungs (kinked endotracheal tube (ETT), patient biting the ETT, secretions in the airway or ETT, etc.). What is a good indicator to actual lung damage is a high plateau pressure. Once you observe a high plateau pressure (> 30 cmH2O), you should immediately switch to pressure control ventilation so you can control the pressures within the patient's lungs instead of forcing a set volume into their lungs and simply accepting the high pressures that their diseased lungs are dictating. Remember, in volume control ventilation, pressure is variable and due to the condition of the patient's lungs. **Healthy lungs report a plateau pressure of < 30 cmH2O while diseased, infected, or significantly injured lungs reflect higher plateau pressures (> 30 cmH2O).**

Plateau pressure indicates that lung damage is occurring. The magnitude of damage is dependent on how high the pressures gets as well as how many breaths are provided. Once we recognize a high plateau pressure, the patient needs to immediately be removed from volume control ventilation and have pressure control ventilation applied. The way to recognize this is to perform an inspiratory hold maneuver and obtain the plateau pressure.

Expiratory Hold Maneuver

The expiratory hold maneuver is performed in <u>pressure control ventilation</u> to identify if auto-PEEP is occurring in the patient's lungs. For multiple reasons, inhaled air can be trapped within a patient's lungs. As gas is forced into a patients lungs, it passes the carina, enters a main bronchus, and approximately 23 divisions later, ends up in an alveoli. During exhalation, gas must find its way out of the lungs before the next inhalation or it becomes trapped. We can cause iatrogenic air trapping (auto-PEEP) by not allowing enough exhalation time (shorter I:E ratios) in patients predisposed to air trapping. COPD, asthma, and pediatric patients all are characterized as having air trapping and so need longer E times to allow time for gases to find their way out of the lung during exhalation.

To perform this maneuver, the 'maneuvers' button is depressed during exhalation (thus prolonging exhalation). The goal of this is to see if there is any excess PEEP than has been set on the ventilator. Most transport ventilators will display "AutoPEEP < 0" if autoPEEP (air trapping) is not occurring. If autoPEEP is present, then the ventilator would display a positive whole number in cmH2O above the set PEEP. If you observe a positive whole number, then you should elongate the expiratory time by changing the I- time to reflect an I:E ratio of 1:4, 1:5, or 1:6. Elongating the E-time allows for more time to exhale, which remedies the air trapping.

### PRACTICE SESSION #8:

1. How can the inspiratory hold maneuver be used as a diagnostic?
2. How can the expiratory hold maneuver be used as a diagnostic?

In summary, the 'maneuvers' feature on a transport ventilator can provide us very important information. With the inspiratory hold maneuver, we can identify the plateau pressure, indicating healthy or diseased lungs. The expiratory hold maneuver alerts us to air trapping. Knowing how to access this information could be vital in the care of your patients.

# 2
# TRANSPORT VENTILATORS

Transport ventilators are fantastic machines that you can utilize to augment pathophysiology and influence it to be closer to normal physiology. That *is* actually what we do at every level of the medical practice, correct? Someone is sick or hurt and we, as medical professionals, step in and apply a therapy to correct their illness or injury. By monitoring and treating derangements in the patient's pulse oximetry and $EtCO2$, we can literally improve the patient's physiology with the mechanical ventilator. That being said, these machines are just that – machines. We can choose and apply settings to the ventilator, but if we ever fail to ensure that our settings are actually being delivered to the patient, then we will never truly be able to harness the power of this machine.

---

**VENT HERO SECRET #7**: Never assume you can seamlessly replicate the settings from a hospital ventilator to a transport ventilator- ever.

---

Consider this call that you may have had before: you arrive at an ICU to pick up a patient and transfer them an hour away by helicopter to a bigger ICU. The patient is on the ventilator, so you dial in your ventilator settings to exactly match what they're currently receiving from the ICU ventilator. From the first moment you apply your transport ventilator, alarms begin sounding in every directions. You examine the ventilator and it reports a 'low minute ventilation' alarm. You review your settings and they exactly match the ICU's ventilator settings. If they match exactly, why in the world is the alarm sounding?

The transport ventilator is much different from a fully programmable hospital ventilator. However there are several similarities. Understanding these differences will allow you to be incredibly successful at operating and troubleshooting the transport ventilator.

Some of the major differences between a hospital ventilator and a transport ventilator are the large number of variables that are precalculated and built into the programming of the transport ventilator. Transport ventilators are not fully programmable like their hospital counterparts. Engineers of transport ventilators build into the programming precalculated variables for purposes of safety and ease of use for the transport clinician. This helps to standardize the care delivered by non–respiratory therapists and non–physicians. The reason for standardization is to remove the numerous calculations that have to be made in order to appropriately mechanically ventilate a patient. In the hospital setting, the respiratory therapist will actually measure multiple variables; that the transport clinician will not even have an opportunity to calculate because several of these variables will have been precalculated.

It's daunting how many calculations a respiratory therapist has to complete before setting up a single patient on the mechanical ventilator. If you want to make yourself as confused and perplexed as possible, then Google 'respiratory therapy calculations' and snatch yourself a .pdf file that is 4-5 pages long filled with mathematical calculations for respiratory therapy. This is why transport ventilators were designed with most of these calculations already done for us. This helps us in that we don't have to calculate every single variable; however, it puts us in a place where if we're not careful, we can get buried in confusing and conflicting information from the transport ventilator.

Ventilator manufacturing companies know you're not a respiratory therapist, so they design and deploy safeguards in the programming of the machine to make it 'easier' on you. In the end, it's actually a convenience because it saves you from an overwhelming number of calculations to endure. That being said, you must learn how to harness this precalculation feature so that you can anticipate problems and issues. For instance, if you set the ventilator to deliver 12 breaths per minute at 500 ccs tidal volume, then the patient's minute ventilation should be 6 liters per minute. If you look at the monitored data on your transport ventilator and the patient is only receiving 4 liters per minute, then you need to investigate why there is a dyssynchrony between the patient and your transport ventilator. We will discuss how to handle such issues in a future chapter.

One of the first things that is precalculated for us is vent tubing, including the length and diameter. Typically, we do not go as transport clinicians and cut certain lengths of tubing or add on extensions like respiratory therapy is trained to do. We simply grab a standard-sized ventilator circuit and attach it to the ventilator. We take for granted that a respiratory therapist has to study for years to be able to coordinate all the variables, including measuring the length of tubing, the diameter of the tubing and multiple other variables that affect how the patient receives the gas the ventilator delivers.

We typically have two options when it comes to choosing ventilator circuits in transport: an adult circuit and a pediatric circuit. Typically, adult circuits are for patients > 20 kg and pediatric circuits are for patients between 5 and 20 kg. What additionally comes into play is the fact that each patient is different and unique. One patient may have longer and larger diameter airway than another. All this effects how much ventilation the patient receives relative to how much is *set* for the patient to receive. We can set certain variables, but they might not be received by the patient. This is why we always strive for a patient-ventilator synchrony and attempt to match our settings to the measured ventilator data that comes from the patient. Once this is achieved, then you will have also achieved patient– ventilator synchrony.

Another important selection made early in mechanical ventilator application is the precalculated patient size: adult, pediatric or infant size. The ventilator precalculates multiple variables into those three age ranges. Normally, the respiratory therapist will calculate the size of the patient and determine how long the vent circuit needs to be and what diameter is appropriate. The transport ventilator, however, has all of this data precalculated and programmed so that when you choose a patient size, these precalculated parameters are applied to the programming. IF you chose the 'adult' size and attempted to apply an infant– sized tidal volume, the transport ventilator would not let you. It would not allow such a low Vt on an adult because it is programmed to recognize an adults normal tidal volume range. At the same time, if you chose an infant size initially, and tried to deliver an adult– sized Vt, it also would not allow you to make that setting.

While this seems incredibly safe and helpful, these precalculations can frequently cause patient–ventilator dyssynchrony in transport medicine. Transport ventilators do a great job of safeguarding our patients from an incorrect setting on the behalf of the transport clinician, but these precalculations also cause confusion and dyssynchrony by increasing the margin of error when initiating and maintaining the mechanical ventilator. Consider a pediatric patient which could range from younger than a toddler all the way to a 17 year old. How then, does one average that broad of a size/ age range? If you choose the pediatric size setting and the patient is a 20 month old, chances are the ventilator will underestimate the patient's true size. In this case, you choose a pediatric setting and calculate the patient needs to be 85 cc of tidal volume. The transport ventilator may assume an average pediatric as being about 10 years old. This would equate to a much larger ventilator tubing for the patient and ultimately result in a exhaled tidal volume that is much less than the set 85 cc for this patient; which is a problem where the set volume isn't reaching the patient's lungs because of the larger ventilator circuit and misleading precalculations.

In summary, there are numerous precalculations that factor into how the transport ventilator interacts with the patient. There are certain safeguards in place, which can sometimes cause patient–ventilator dyssynchrony by over or under–estimating the actual patient size. It is the goal of this text to train the transport clinician to appropriately set the transport ventilator, but to synchronize and maintain the transport ventilator on all patient types and conditions based on clinical observations. In future chapters of this text, we will examine how to best plan to prevent ventilator dyssynchrony, how to detect patient–ventilator dyssynchrony, and how to troubleshoot dyssynchrony once it is discovered.

## PRACTICE SESSION #9:

1. Describe how a transport ventilator is different from a hospital ventilator.
2. Will applying an ICU ventilator's settings to your transport ventilator without alarms sounding be common? Explain.

# 3
# VENTILATOR STRATEGIES

It is often asked of me to lecture on specific ventilator strategies. I want to make something clear-strategies are simply templates to help you remember how to INITIALLY apply the mechanical ventilator to a patient. These strategies are based on current conditions of the patient.  In theory standardized strategies seem like good ideas, but why learn strategies when you can just learn a universal approach that almost targets any type of patient? We will soon discuss a universal approach to the mechanical ventilator that derives its specific ventilator settings based on the patient's pH status. For instance, if a patient is acidotic, then you'll need a larger than normal minute ventilation to ensure you're getting rid of the appropriate amount of acid from the respiratory system (in the form of $CO_2$).  Most of the standardized strategies help you memorize respiratory rate and tidal volume range. Why learn five (or more) different strategies when you can simply learn a universal approach to the ventilator?

So if one should avoid using standardized strategies, why were strategies developed? Ventilator strategies were developed, as previously mentioned, so that a basic template can be applied based on multiple patient types and conditions. The clinicians auditing charts of ventilated patients discovered other clinicians were not applying the appropriate settings nor making appropriate ventilator changes based on the patient's vital signs and monitored ventilator data. Undoubtedly, these reviewing well-versed clinicians developed templates for the less savvy clinicians to follow, in order to assist them in correctly utilizing the mechanical ventilator.

This chapter will describe a selection of common ventilator strategies. We will not need to practice these strategies, because we will soon unveil a simple universal approach to mechanical ventilation. However, it is important for you to be aware of these strategies.

It is also important to mention that the strategies below are provided using tidal volumes, however, you can easily transfer these strategies into pressure control ventilation. To accomplish this you simply set the pressure control setting, monitor Vte, and titrate the PC setting to target a Vte within the ventilator strategy's tidal volume range. Remember, that you can still nearly-control tidal volume with pressure control ventilation, but you just have to titrate the PC setting to reach the desired Vt (which is indicated by the Vte).

## Standard Strategy

The standard strategy (adult) is for patients with healthy lungs and airways. These patients could include those who have overdosed on a drug or medication, hypotensive trauma patients (without damage to the lungs or airways), and medical patients without lung or airway pathophysiology.

Respiratory Rate: 10-14 breaths/min

Tidal Volume: 6-8 cc/kg of IBW

PEEP: 3-5 cmH2O

I:E: 1:2

FiO2: 1.0

## Minute Ventilation Supportive Strategy

This strategy was designed for patients with sepsis, acidosis, or any other condition characterized by a hypermetabolic state (increased metabolism). With high metabolic states, there will be an increase in acid in in the blood which is converted to $CO_2$ for removal. This strategy allows for an increased minute ventilation so that acid (in the form of $CO_2$) can be displaced from the body by patient's respiratory system.

Respiratory Rate: 15-20 breaths/min

Tidal Volume: 8-10 cc/kg of IBW

PEEP: 3-5 cmH2O

I:E: 1:2

FiO2: 1.0

Key Features: higher respiratory rates and tidal volumes ultimately increase the minute ventilation needed by these patients to clear out enough acid from the body and correct acidosis.


## PRACTICE SESSION #10:

1. Describe how to initiate mechanical ventilation on a patient without pulmonary pathophysiology and with normal hemodynamics.
2. Your patient is a DKA patient with a pH of 7.3. Describe how to initiate mechanical ventilation on this patient.


## Flow Supportive Strategy

This strategy is specific for patients who present with any pathophysiology that is consistent with air-trapping. This would include patients with asthma, COPD, and anaphylaxis. Additionally, smaller pediatric patients will benefit from this strategy because they have an immature respiratory system and their pulmonary tissue will not expel air out of the lungs during exhalation quickly, which causes air-trapping.

Respiratory Rate:8-10 breaths/min

Tidal Volume: 7-8 cc/kg of IBW

PEEP: 3-4 cmH2O

I:E: 1:4, 1:5, or 1:6

FiO2: 1.0

Key Features: lower respiratory rates allow for more exhalation time and setting an I:E ratio with a larger (or longer) E-time also ensures longer periods the patient can exhale and release trapped air. The goal is to prevent air-trapping.

## Neuroprotective Strategy

Historically, patients that have experienced a head injury or stroke were ventilated based on a neuroprotective strategy. The premise is to prevent increased intrathoracic pressures by reducing (or limiting) PEEP. Increased PEEP (> 8cmH2O) will tamponade the delicate alveolar capillaries which are not physiologically exposed to PEEPs over 5 cmH2O. When you apply this tamponade effect across both lungs, you get a significant reduction in cardiac output as the PEEP prevents the forward flow of blood. This causes a back pressure of blood, much like CHF, and therefore blood backs up into both superior and inferior vena cavae. As blood continues to back up the superior vena cava, it will end up in the cranium, which can increase ICP and therefore cause secondary brain injury. This mechanism is currently out of vogue as the medical literature has failed to provide strong evidence to its validity or benefit them.

Respiratory Rate: 10-14 breaths/min

Tidal Volume: 7-8 cc/kg of IBW

PEEP: Keep under 8 cmH2O to prevent an ↑ in ICP

I:E: 1:2

FiO2: 1.0

Key Features: this strategy prevents higher PEEPs, which at one time was thought to both reduce cardiac output (still believed to be true) and increase ICP (no longer strongly supported).


## PRACTICE SESSION #11:

1. Describe how to initiate mechanical ventilation on a patient exhibiting a closed head injury and increased ICP.
2. Your patient is an asthmatic and has been self-medicating for 24 hours and now requires intubation. Describe how to initiate mechanical ventilation on this patient.


## Lung Protective Strategies

Any patient who presents with damaged (from trauma) or diseased lungs, has been traditionally targeted with the lung protective ventilator strategy. This strategy is ideal for patients with acute respiratory distress syndrome (ARDS) or acute lung injury (ALI). Patients within these categories would include patients with burned respiratory tracts, atelectasis, aspiration pneumonia, or in the event caustic substances have entered the airway.

Respiratory Rate: 18-22 breaths/min

Tidal Volume: 6-7 cc/kg of IBW

<u>PEEP</u>: 5

<u>I:E</u>: 1:2

<u>FiO2</u>: 1.0

<u>Key Features</u>: by reducing the tidal volume and increasing respiratory rate you can prevent dangerous plateau pressures (the true indicator of current lung injury) while maintaining the physiologically demanded minute ventilation.

## Hypotensive Strategy

While I am not a big fan of ventilator strategies, I do like this one. The premise of this strategy is to minimize the number of times the lungs fill up with air. The designers of this strategy realized that with inhalation comes a tamponade effect, similar to the neuroprotective strategy. When patients already have low blood pressure, we want to prevent any further drop in blood pressure. To accomplish this, we increase the tidal volume (or pressure control if in pressure control ventilation) and reduce the respiratory rate. This way, we reduce the number of time the tamponade effect occurs, and therefore reduce reductions in blood pressure caused by inhalation. As you adjust the RR and Vt, make sure to target a minute ventilation that matched what the patient was breathing prior to your adjustments.

<u>Respiratory Rate</u>: 8-10 breaths/min

<u>Tidal Volume</u>: 10-12 cc/kg of IBW

<u>PEEP</u>: 3-5

<u>I:E</u>: 1:2

<u>FiO2</u>: 1.0
The
<u>Key Features</u>: reduces the number of times we apply a tamponade

to a patient during inspiration (lower respiratory rates). We can increase the tidal volume (assuming we do not breech plateau pressures of > 30 cmH2O) to meet the physiologically demanded minute ventilation.

## PRACTICE SESSION #12:

1. Describe how to initiate mechanical ventilation on a patient with low blood pressure.
2. Your patient has ARDS. Describe how to initiate mechanical ventilation on this patient.

Somewhere along the way, some savvy clinicians created a template for how to handle different patient conditions using the mechanical ventilator. However, from our investigation of minute ventilation, we already know how important it is to target a minute ventilation based on the patient's condition. So why do we need to memorize multiple different strategies when we can derive the initial settings from simple data obtained from the patient? Ultimately, we don't need multiple templates. We really need to fortify our knowledge, practice, and skill on a universal critical care transport ventilator approach.

Challenge accepted.

# 4
## THE UNIVERSAL VENTILATOR APPROACH

Over the last decade, I have strung together a multitude of clinical pearls regarding the mechanical ventilator. The mechanical ventilator, and specifically those designed for transport, is not an enigma. It can be tamed, but it will require you to be clinically open minded. You'll need to discard some conventions you've come to memorize and hold as gospel. If you can accept these challenges, then you'll find and much more practical and user-friendly method to applying mechanical ventilator than you've ever seen before. I will now show you a revolutionary way of utilizing this powerful device.

## A LESSON ON THE IMPORTANCE OF PERFUSION

A redneck nurse, paramedic, AND pharmacist once asked why it took so long to teach a CPR class? I insisted that the American Heart Association set the time scales. He claimed that he could teach the class in about 15 seconds. He told me, "Air goes in and out, and blood goes around and around. If they ain't doing it, then you gotta. They're 'posed' to match".

Seems too simplistic, doesn't it? Well, he is exactly right. Our entire job as critical care transport clinicians is to deliver oxygen to the patient's tissues and prevent acidosis. That is all we are required to do. Consider a patient who has overdosed on a narcotic. It will be our role to ensure an open airway where we can administer high flow oxygen into the lungs. Once we achieve a high oxygen content within the alveoli, we then need to push that oxygen (which at this point has attached to a red blood cell) around the vasculature where it will be a offloaded within a tissue bed. From there, the oxygen will find its way into a cell where it can unite with glucose to generate energy, heat, water, and carbon dioxide ($CO_2$). Our role is to ultimately facilitate metabolism because in doing so we prevent acidosis.

Given the gravity of our roles as defenders of acidosis, it is incredibly important we quickly identify and correct any hypotension. If blood pressure isn't high enough to perfuse distal tissues (aka end organs, aka heart, brain, lungs, skin, liver, etc.) then we are failing to support the second part of the "redneck perfusion equation" of 'air in and out must match the blood going around and around'. Without ensuring an adequate amount oxygenated red blood cells are being transported to the tissues for oxygen offload, then we fall short on the right side of the redneck perfusion equation: 'blood goes around and around.' To illustrate this point, consider minute ventilation. In an adult, normal minute ventilation is 4-8 L/min (this represents the air in and out). Normal cardiac output for an adult is 5-6 L/min (represents the blood going around and around). See how they are damn near identical? Oh my, that redneck was right!

We must, therefore, be diligent in identifying and correcting any hypotension. One of the first questions I want answered very early upon arrival to the scene or at the patient's bedside in a  hospital is 'what is their hemodynamic status?' What I'm really asking is 'what is their blood pressure and is it producing a palpable distal pulse'. I almost could care less what the numerical systolic and diastolic blood pressure are because what matters most importantly is if the patient's cardiac output is producing a pulse or not. I will clinically classify the pulse as strong, weak but present, or absent. Once I identify that a pulse is either weak or absent, I initiate aggressive fluid resuscitation and prepare for pressors, should the patient warrant them. I will routinely reach down and feel the patient's radial pulse to obtain a qualitative trend on their perfusion. Once I feel a strong pulse transition to a 'weak but present' pulse, then I quickly manage it.

It is imperative that we quickly address any hypotension because without a perfusing blood pressure, we cannot trust pulse oximetry and EtCO2 data. Consider a patient who just became hypotensive. As they breathe, oxygen is delivered to the red blood cell, but never makes it to the tissues because the pressure isn't great enough to push blood all the way to the capillaries of a tissue. If oxygen is not arriving at a tissue, then it can never enter a cell and ultimately prevent acidosis, therefore, acids are created from anaerobic metabolism. Additionally, if the blood pressure is not sufficient to get oxygen to the tissues, then it also is insufficient to remove CO2 from the cells for delivery to the lungs so it can be exhaled. If we were to obtain blood samples on this hypothetical patient over time we would see a lowering pH (becoming more acidic) and a decreasing CO2 (because it is stuck in the cells and not yet in the blood stream where we obtain labs from). Within the cells, acid and CO2 continue to build up towards dangerous levels. Once perfusion is restored, all that acid and CO2 is released into the blood stream. Lowering pH would be observed as well as an increase in CO2 (from all the CO2 being released from the cells).

The bottom line is this: you will not be able to trust the values normally used to make ventilator changes unless you achieve and maintain perfusion of the distal tissues. Therefore, be aggressive and initiate fluid resuscitation (including blood if indicated) and pressors (if the patient warrants it) early in your treatment to ensure the SpO2 and EtCO2 data you obtain is accurate.

> **VH Rule #8:** low blood pressure provides unreliable EtCO2 and SpO2 values.

## PRACTICE SESSION #13:

1. Explain why perfusion is important to the mechanically ventilated patient.
2. How can low perfusion and blood pressure affect the EtCO2 and SpO2?

## ACIDOSIS AND MINUTE VENTILATION

As mentioned, minute ventilation is very important to the transport ventilator clinician. Minute ventilation dictates the values of pCO2 and EtCO2. Measuring either EtCO2 or pCO2 will provide a close estimate of the patient's pH status, which is what physicians use to make ventilator changes. Rarely in transport medicine will we have the luxury of ABG data, so we must practice using EtCO2 to guide our ventilator changes.

When considering settings for mechanical ventilation with a transport ventilator, there traditionally have been two schools of thought. The first, and still the most common, is to apply ventilator default settings or settings based on a standardized strategy (see chapter 3). This seems like an inefficient methodology because if these settings are incorrect, you could be busy awhile finding the right combination of ventilator changes to arrive at the 'Goldie Locks' type of settings where they are "just right" for the patient. The second school of thought is to utilize the strategies discussed in chapter 3. As previously voiced, why memorize 5-6 strategies when studying just one that is flexible adequately achieves our clinical goals?

I offer a third school of thought, which targets a selected minute ventilation based on the patient's pH status. If the patient is known to have acidosis (low pH) or is suspected of having acidosis, then we simply choose a minute ventilation to be delivered that is just outside the patient's normal minute ventilation range. If there is no evidence to support an acidotic condition, then it is reasonable to choose a minute ventilation within the normal range for the patient's age range.

### Normal Minute Ventilation Ranges (by age group):
1. **Adults: 4-8 L/min**
2. **Peds: 2-4 L/min**
3. **Infant: 1-2 L/min**

Why should you utilize and practice this methodology? Consider a patient in diabetic ketoacidosis (DKA). These patients do not have enough insulin to force glucose into the cells (out of the vascular system). This causes acidosis within the cells as metabolism progresses in the form of anaerobic metabolism. To add insult to injury, their body then breaks down other macromolecules (specifically fats) to liberate more energy and with it more acid is released. There should be no question that these patients are acidotic. They usually present with altered mental status, elevated blood glucose, and increased respiratory rate. Human pathophysiology dictates an increased respiratory rate and depth in times of acidosis to help 'blow off' $CO_2$ which the body generates to get rid of excess acid. Adults experiencing DKA can have respiratory rates of 30 or more and above normal tidal volumes. If an adult patient is breathing 32 bpm with 500 cc of tidal volume (a very conservative tidal volume in these patients) then their physiology is demanding 16 L/min of minute ventilation to clear out enough acid to prevent cell death. Recall that the body can take acid and convert it into water and $CO_2$. Therefore, in acidic conditions the body will attempt to increase respiratory rate and depth to exhale as much $CO_2$ as possible because that is the equivalent of exhaling acid. If you arrive and apply ventilator default settings of RR 12 and Vt 500 (minute ventilation of 6 L/min) on this DKA patient, then you could kill them by preventing them from clearing out just the right amount of acid (in the form of $CO_2$) which would quickly cause ventricular fibrillation and death.

To identify the patient's acidotic status, I suggest keeping it simple. With three pieces of information you can identify whether a patient is acidotic or not, and which will allow you to select the appropriate minute ventilation for your patient. The first of these questions is the most sensitive to acid status and the third being only suggestive of acidosis. I know that sounds confusing and unclear, so let's just go ahead and take a look at these three questions to help rule in or rule out acidosis.

1.  **Does the patient have a low pH?**
2.  **Is the patient breathing really fast?**
3.  **Does the patient have a high EtCO2?**

These questions will provide insight to the pH status of your patient. The question, "Does the patient have a low pH?" is very simple to answer if you have a recent (within 30 minutes or so) ABG. This can be obtained from the sending facility or a venous blood gas (VBG) can be obtained from an iStat if you have that piece of equipment on hand. The VBG has been described in the medical literature as being correlative to ABG except in shock states, where it is not well studied. ABGs are always more sensitive for ventilation and oxygenation decision making. The pH is the principal value that detects whether your patient is acidotic, alkalotic, or is pH neutral. If the pH is less than 7.35, then the patient is acidotic.

The second question, "Is the patient breathing really fast?" identifies if there is a pathophysiology consistent with mass offloading $CO_2$ to reduce tissue and serum acids. It helps us identity a metabolic acidosis issue, or at least heavily suggests it. That's all you need is a suggestion that the patient is acidotic. Once you observe significant tachypnea and suspect acidosis, then you can safely choose a minute ventilation just outside the normal range for your patient. Now, tachypnea is a poor diagnostic symptom, but when tachypnea is higher than 10 more respirations per minute (greater than the highest normal value for the patient's age range), it is similar to Kussmaul's respirations, which we see in severe metabolic states. So, if a patient is breathing similar to Kussmaul's (greater than 30/min for adults) then it is reasonable to consider it is because of acidosis and therefore we need to set a higher than normal minute ventilation. For instance, if your adult patient ingested antifreeze, then you would expect metabolic acidosis with faster respiratory rates as the body tries to clear out acid. In this case, instead of applying the ventilator to deliver a minute ventilation of 4-8 L/min (normal range for an adult), choosing 9 or 10 L/min as the minute ventilation would be better suited to manage acidosis than the normal range.

The third question to assist you in identifying potential acidosis is, "Does the patient have a high EtCO2?" If the patient has an elevated EtCO2, then it could possibly be because of an acidotic condition. Elevated EtCO2 is only potential evidence of acidosis, whereas a low pH is actual evidence. A patient breathing significantly fast (> 10 than above the highest normal respirations per minute) is somewhere between these evidence strengths. I like to think of these strengths in this manner: low pH is actual evidence, significant tachypnea is strongly suggestive evidence, and elevated EtCO2 is only potential evidence. If any of these questions are answered with a 'yes', then apply a minute ventilation of 9 to 10 L/min, which is just outside the range of normal (for an adult) by an increase of 1-2 L/min.

Adding 1-2 L/min to the upper value of normal for minute ventilation is a rule I call **Swearingen's Rule**, because, well I came up with it. Once your initial settings are set, you still have to let the EtCO2 confirm if the initial minute ventilation setting is correct or if other changes need to be made.

Remember, setting the mechanical ventilator has historically been arbitrary for transport clinicians. We would adopt the default settings or settings that were already on a hospital ventilator and then maintain these settings the most part. Here we are simply suggesting choosing minute ventilations that are barely outside the patient's normal range in the face of acidosis. We are currently engaging in research that will help identify if there is a 'magic number' or optimal range as a starting point for minute ventilation in the face of acidosis. In the end, choosing the appropriate minute ventilation is an educated guess which, if appropriate, can prevent your patient from becoming increasingly and dangerously acidotic. I am suggesting here to investigate these questions and let them help you decide to initiate mechanical ventilation within the normal range (if no acidosis suspected) or follow Swearingen's Rule and apply 1-2 L/min beyond the normal range (if acidosis suspected).

---

**<u>VH Rule #9</u>: Stop guessing on minute ventilation. Start using the information the patient provides you.**

---

58

1. Your patient is a 9 year old trauma patient. What is the typical minute ventilation of a patient this age?
2. List the three questions needed to identify whether a patient is acidotic.


DERIVING INITIAL VENTILATOR SETTINGS

The third major concept that needs to be addressed when applying the mechanical ventilator to the patient is patient/ventilator synchrony. To achieve this, we first need to apply appropriate ventilator settings and then double check to ensure what we have set is actually reaching the patient. One incredibly common failure in our field is the initiation of mechanical ventilation using default settings and then never obtaining confirmation data from the vent that the settings are actually reaching the patient. It is a real situation where you may choose the default settings of RR 12 and have Vt 500 (minute ventilation is therefore 6 L/min), but the ventilator 'low minute ventilation' alarm is sounding and displaying only 3 L/min is reaching the patient. How can this be? It's because there is a dyssynchrony between the patient and the ventilator. Spoiler: this is an easy thing to identify, but you need to be aggressive in looking for it once you first apply the mechanical ventilator.

---

**VH Rule #10**: **Never assume your settings are reaching the patient. Prove to yourself the desired settings are reaching the patient.**

---

In the upcoming pages, we will discuss not only how to arrive at appropriate ventilator settings, but also how to prove to yourself (and whoever may read your patient's chart) that the settings you applied were reaching the patient.

Selecting Calculated Initial Ventilator Settings

I will now present a series of calculations resulting in a respiratory rate and tidal volume that targets a specific minute ventilation for a particular patient. This takes the guess-work out of choosing initial ventilator settings and replaces it with settings that are appropriate for a particular patient's condition. This makes much more sense than guessing or using the ventilator's default settings followed by too long of a time adjusting the ventilator during transport.

Once you have identified your target minute ventilation, you need to choose how to deliver it. Recall that minute ventilation is the respiratory rate multiplied by the tidal volume [VE = Vt x RR]. Using this equation, deriving the RR and Vt should be easy. Tidal volumes can vary, but when it varies too much the patient either can be hypoventilated or can suffer lung injury from barotrauma. For this reason, I like to calculate the patient's ideal body weight (IBW) and then calculate what I call the ideal tidal volume (IVt). The IVt is the tidal volume specific for that patient, and when divided into the chosen minute ventilation, provides us with the respiratory rate needed to meet that minute ventilation.

Let's look at an example. Consider the adult patient presented earlier in the text that was suffering from DKA. He is breathing 32 breaths/min. We assess his condition to be highly suggestive of acidosis, therefore, we apply a minute ventilation of 9 L/min based on Swearingen's Rule (8 L/min + 1 L/min = 9 L/min). Next, we need to calculate the person's ideal body weight (IBW). The Devine formula is current and widely accepted formula for IBW:

**IBW = (2.3)(pt height over 60 inches) + (50 for males or 45.5 for females)**

If our patient is 6'0" and male, then they are 12 inches over 5 feet (5 feet = 60 inches). Therefore, (2.3 x 12) + (50) = 77.6 kg is the ideal body weight. Then, we take their IBW and multiply it by the normal factor for tidal volume, which is 5-8 cc/kg. I usually use 6 or 7 as the tidal volume factor because it this is the middle range of normal. Calculating this, we arrive at (77.6) x (7 cc/kg) = 543.2 cc as the ideal tidal volume. Finally, we can divide this ideal tidal volume into the targeted minute ventilation on this patient which yields (9000cc/ 543.2 cc) = 16.5, or 17. So, to deliver 9 L/min (or 9000 cc/min) on this patient we need to apply a Vt of 543 cc and a RR of 17.

Now, if you are choosing to set the patient on pressure control ventilation instead of volume control ventilation (in the above example), you can still target a minute ventilation, but as we have previously mentioned you cannot directly change the tidal volume. To effect a change in tidal volume while utilizing pressure control ventilation you must change the pressure control setting and monitor the exhaled tidal volume (Vte), which is data measured by the ventilator and displayed to the clinician. So, if we continue with the previous example, you would set your ventilator to deliver a RR of 17 and a pressure control (PC) of 20 cmH2O. To achieve your target minute ventilation of 9 L/min, you'll need to monitor Vte. If you observe a Vte of 625 cc, then you would need to reduce the PC setting. Small changes provide better feedback than big changes, so it is wise to change the PC from 20 cmH2O to 18 cmH2O. Let's say this dropped the Vte to 575 cc. This means we need to reduce PC again. This time we reduce the PC to 16 cmH2O which results in our Vte reducing to 540 cc. This is extremely close to our ideal tidal volume. Therefore, if we keep the pressure control setting (which is achieving the ideal tidal volume) and maintain the calculated RR of 17, then we will successfully be achieving our target minute ventilation of 9 L/min.

If you <u>understand</u> these concepts, but do not <u>practice</u> them then prepare to fail. It is necessary to not only understand but to practice to ensure success at the patient's bedside during real life patient scenarios. This is a skill, and it needs to be practiced. As a US National Paralympic Volleyball player, I have to practice. If I reduce my practice times by half each week, my practice efforts simply maintain my current skills. If I double my normal practice time, I not only maintain my abilities but can also improve upon my current abilities. Using this calculation technique for arriving at a RR and Vte from a targeted minute ventilation also takes practice. Dedicate some good practice time towards its mastery.

## Calculations to Complete:
1. **Calculate IBW**
    a. [(2.3)(pt ht > 60 inches) + (50 for male, 45.5 for female)]
    b. Peds: 8 + (age in years x 2)
    c. Infant: (9 + months in age) / 2
2. **Calculate ITV**
    a. 5-8 cc/kg
    b. Multiply this factor by the IBW
3. **Calculate RR**
    a. Divide desired VE by the IVT


## PRACTICE SESSION #15:

1. Calculate the IBW, ITV, and RR of a patient who is 6'4", male, and who needs a VE of 11 L/min.
2. Calculate the IBW, ITV, and RR of a patient who is 5'7", female, and who needs a VE of 7 L/min.
3. Calculate the IBW, ITV, and RR of a patient who is 6'1", male, and who needs a VE of 8 L/min.


Selecting Non-Calculated Initial Ventilator Settings

Once you have calculated the RR and Vt (or Vte in pressure control mode) based on a targeted minute ventilation, then you need to select the final initial ventilator settings that do not require calculating. These settings include the I:E ratio, FiO2, PEEP, and pressure support (if in SIMV). You may be thinking, "I:E is a calculated setting," but I would argue with this line of thinking. You simply need to adjust the I time to achieve an I:E ratio of 1:2 (if an adult patient has no bronchospasm pathophysiology) or 1:4-1:6 (in small pediatric patients or in patients with bronchospasm/air trapping of any etiology). In the transport environment with a transport ventilator it is not necessary to calculate I-times or E-times, but more importantly to monitor the I:E ratio.

Next, you would want to choose an appropriate PEEP setting. Normal physiologic PEEP is 2-5 cmH2O. When a critical care transport team is called upon, it is reasonable to assume the patient is acutely ill or injured, and therefore, I choose a PEEP on the high side of the normal range (usually 4-5 cmH2O of PEEP). This approach ensures a higher amount of oxygen crossing the alveolar capillary membrane than would occur with a lower PEEP. We can always titrate down the PEEP and FiO2 if the patient maintains high pulse oximetry or PaO2 (per ABG).

The fraction of inspired oxygen (FiO2) setting is normally set to 1.0 (or 100% oxygen) at the initial application of the ventilator. Just like PEEP, this setting can be titrated down should the patient's pulse oximetry and/or PaO2 remain high. It is imperative to keep in mind that the only two effective ways of improving oxygenation (measured by SpO2) is with either PEEP or FiO2. We will discuss more on ventilator changes in an upcoming section (see Surfing EtCO2 and SpO2, page 69).

Finally, if you are using the SIMV mode, you can decide to set a pressure support (PS). As previously mentioned, PS is only brought into play when the patient is allowed by the SIMV mode to inspire on their own power. When the patient is allowed to inspire on his own, you as the clinician can decide to help them out with a 'turbo boost' (PS of 10 cmH2O is a common starting point) or you can set the PS to zero cmH2O and let the patient inspire completely on their own. The normal range for PS is 5 cmH2o to 20 cmH2O.

### Non- Calculation Settings to Select
1. I:E Ratio
    a. 1:2 for non-bronchospastic lungs and non- infants
    b. 1:4- 1:6 for infants and in patients with air trapping/ bronchospasm
2. FiO2
    a. Initially set at 1.0 (100%)
    b. Titrate down in increments of 0.1 as long as the pulse oximetry remains over 95%.

3. PEEP
    a. Initially set between 2-5 cmH2O
    b. Increase to improve oxygenation.
4. Pressure Support
    a. Initially set 5-10 cmH2O
    b. Increasing will increase VE and can decrease EtCO2

## PRACTICE SESSION #16:

1. Determine the I:E ratio, FiO2, and PEEP on the following patient: 4 month old with pneumonia.
2. Determine the I:E ratio, FiO2, and PEEP on the following patient: 35 y/o trauma patient with hypoxia and hypotension.
3. Determine the I:E ratio, FiO2, and PEEP on the following patient: 21 y/o exhibiting shortness of breath and wheezes.

## ENSURE PATIENT/ VENTILATOR SYNCHRONY

I have a question: Have you ever treated someone for hypoglycemia? I am sure you have. Once glucose has been administered to the patient, how do you know it worked? A repeat glucose check would reveal a corrected or a persistently low blood glucose. Therefore double checking your work is very important. Then why would anyone ever apply settings on a ventilator to mechanically ventilate a patient and FAIL to review the monitored data provided by the ventilator? It doesn't make sense, but this happens frequently in the field.

Once initial settings are applied to the ventilator and applied to the patient, it is imperative to be able to prove that the settings are actually reaching the patient's lungs. If we fail to ensure our settings are reaching the patient, we could quite possibly be faced with patient-ventilator dyssynchrony. This limits the power and benefit of the ventilator if the settings never reach the patient. There are five different monitored data points that are important to routinely utilize to ensure your settings match what the patient is actually experiencing.

**VH Rule #11**: If you fail to ensure that what you set is reaching the patient, then you ensure ventilator failure.

Remember Minute Ventilation

The minute ventilation is the prime factor when deciding on appropriate settings because it is directly related to the patient's pH status. Remember, physicians use the pH in their clinical decision-making in ventilator management. It is important to not only set an appropriate minute ventilation, but also to confirm that the set (expected) minute ventilation is reaching the patient.

To ensure minute ventilation you need to observe the ventilator's monitored data display. Let us assume you are targeting a minute ventilation of 6 L/min by setting a RR of 12 and a Vt of 500cc (12 x 500 is 6000cc, or 6 L). You reach to the ventilator and set the RR to 12 and the Vt to 500cc. However, just because you made these setting selections does not mean the patient is actually receiving them. It is imperative to obtain a 'pulse check' on what the ventilator is actually doing. This can be accomplished by observing the monitored data display panel for the VE, which the ventilator calculates from frequency (f) and the exhaled tidal volume (Vte). The VE observed on the display panel is the ACTUAL minute ventilation the patient is experiencing and therefore should be trusted over any expected minute ventilation calculations done with the RR and Vt settings. The main concept is simple- trust the measured data from the vent and not the expected calculations. The ventilator is a machine and if we just assume that the patient is experiencing the settings we set then we are blinding ourselves to what may actually be occurring. We must always double check the settings we apply to ensure it is actually reaching our patients.

**Minute Ventilation Check:**

**Set**: RR and Vt (targeting a specific minute ventilation)
**Check**: VE on the monitored data display
**VE Lower than Expected**: investigate f and Vte

If the measured VE is less than the expected VE, you will need to investigate frequency and exhaled minute ventilation to identify which is the culprit. Because VE = f x Vte, then one of the two has to be the reason for the VE variation from the expected minute ventilation. Because the lung is a closed system, you will rarely ever observe more volume coming out of a set of lungs (Vte) than the ventilator was set to deliver (Vt).

**Respiratory Rate Check:**

**Set**: RR
**Check**: frequency (f)
**Frequency HIGHER than the preset RR:** Sedate the patient and/or increase the sensitivity setting.

There are 2 major reasons that the frequency (f) will be larger than the preset RR: 1) too low sensitivity setting, and 2) an awake or waking patient. In a flight scenario there will be vibrations in your aircraft, and these vibrations can trigger breaths if the sensitivity setting is too low. Recall that the sensitivity setting is a whole number (negative) whose units are in cmH2O. A higher sensitivity makes it more difficult for a patient to trigger a breath because it requires more negative pressure to trigger that breath. So, to reduce the number of breaths triggered by vibrations, set the sensitivity at higher settings.

The other reason for a higher frequency other than a preset RR is the simple fact that the patient maybe waking up and overbreathing the ventilator. Once the frequency begins to increase away from the preset RR, assuming the sensitivity is set to its highest setting, then assume the patient is waking up from previous sedation. Closely monitoring the frequency can be an early diagnostic alerting you to an awakening patient. Once you identify an increased frequency relative to the preset RR, then apply appropriate sedation or paralytics to ensure the patient isn't overbreathing the ventilator.

There is a school of thought where some clinicians want to keep the patient's inherent and pre-intubation RR, but this is more of a protective measure to prevent the inexperienced ventilator clinician from applying a minute ventilation that is too low. As long as you are providing the appropriate minute ventilation, then you can take over complete control of their respiratory effort and vary RR from their inherent and pre- intubation RR. How do you know if your minute ventilation is appropriate? Target an $EtCO2$ of 35-45 mmHg (or as close as possible). The $EtCO2$ is closely related to the patient's pH, and therefore can be utilized and trusted to make ventilator-based clinical decisions. If we apply an appropriate minute ventilation guided by the patient's $EtCO2$, then we can safely deviate from the patient's inherent and /or pre-intubation RR.

### Tidal Volume Check:

**Set**: Vt
**Check**: Exhaled tidal volume (Vte)
**Vte Lower than set Vt**: Increase the Vt to overcome
    dead space.

If the measured Vte is lower than the set Vt, then you most likely have a smaller air leak or a dead space problem. It would have to be a smaller air leak because a large air leak would not allow the ventilator circuit to pressurize and it would give a low pressure alarm. A small air leak would allow the vent circuit to pressurize but would prevent the full preset tidal volume to reach the patient, which results in a lower Vte than the set Vt.

A dead space problem is different. Recall these transport ventilators are different from standard hospital ventilators because they precalculate several measurements that hospital vents do not. There are standard tubing lengths and sizes, there are standard patient sizes (infant, pediatric, adult), and several others. When a specific patient varies greatly from these standard sizes, we can find significant clinical differences. If you have preset a patient to receive a tidal volume of

500 cc and they only receive 300 cc (less than 50cc of difference is acceptable), there is most likely a leak or dead space problem. Since, we cannot do much about a leak other than ensure our endotracheal tube cuff has a good seal, we can assume a dead space problem.

To correct a dead space problem, we need to increase our preset Vt to overcome the dead space. For instance, if we preset 500 cc and our measured Vte is only 300 cc, then adding the difference of 200 is a good starting point to make up the dead space. Therefore, we would increase the preset Vt from 500 cc to 700 cc (500 cc + 200 cc = 700 cc). The danger here would be in the form of peak inspiratory pressure (PIP) becoming too high with this increase in volume, so simply keep an eye on PIP for the first few breaths at the higher Vt setting of 700 cc. As long as the PIP remains under 40 cmH2O there isn't much danger of damaging the lung. Keep in mind your Vte is what the patient is ACTUALLY receiving. As you increase your delivered tidal volume, the only volume actually reaching your patient is the Vte, and not the Vt. **Upon arrival to a receiving facility if someone challenges you as to why you have such a high vent setting, professionally remind them that you are targeting a specific Vte and the increased Vt setting is being utilized as a tool to overcome the dead space assisting you to achieve a specific Vte.**

## PRACTICE SESSION #17:

1. Your expected VE is 6 L/min and the ventilator is displaying a VE of 3 L/min. What should you investigate next?
2. You are troubleshooting a high minute ventilation alarm and note a RR of 16, VE of 9 L/min, and f of 22. What needs to be done to correct the high minute ventilation alarm?
3. You have set the ventilator to deliver a Vt of 550 and it only delivers 501. Does this represent a significant dead space problem?.

## Peak Inspiratory Pressure (PIP) Check:

**Set**: Not a setting- it's measured from the ventilator.
**Check**: PIP
**PIP > 35 cmHg**: Correct DOPE causes. If no cause found, proceed to check plateau pressure.

If the PIP is larger than 35 mmHg, then there is a chance that the lung is experiencing damage. PIP doesn't confirm lung damage, but rather suggests it. Once there is a high PIP, we need to look into possible etiologies and spot correct them.

The DOPE acronym is a useful tool to rule out these potential etiologies. The 'D' in DOPE stands for dislodgement. As the endotracheal tube (ETT) accidentally is extubated it can land against the back of the oropharynx, which occludes the end of the ETT and is recorded as increased PIP. Confirm the ETT has not migrated to rule out dislodgement as a cause of high PIP.

The 'O' in the DOPE acronym stands for obstruction. The ventilator circuit itself includes the patient's lungs. Anything within the circuit that reduces air flow will increase airway pressures and results in a high PIP alarm. Kinking of the endotracheal tube or ventilator circuit, foreign material, secretions, and a coughing patient can all cause an obstruction in the airway. Ensuring all tubes are not kinked and suctioning the airway should rule out most of these etiologies. If the patient is coughing, then consider sedation.

The 'P' in the DOPE acronym stands for pneumothorax, and specifically it refers to a tension pneumothorax. This is also an obstruction problem, but it is used on its own for purposes of having a functioning acronym (DOPE). With a tension pneumothorax, there are great pressures in the thorax and these pressures prevent air from being advanced into the lungs. Be sure to look for signs and symptoms of a tension pneumothorax and decompress as soon as one is identified.

The 'E' in the DOPE acronym stands for equipment. This is the concept that helps remind you to check to ensure all of your equipment is applied correctly. If vent circuit tubes are flip-flopped or if someone is standing on the vent circuit then increased PIPs will be registered.

Ultimately, there are mechanical, anatomical, and physiological reasons that can cause a high PIP alarm to go be set off. The DOPE acronym is a template to help you recall some of these etiologies. Once you have identified one, correct it. Finally, if you cannot identify the cause for an increased PIP, proceed to obtaining a plateau pressure.

### Plateau Pressure (Pplat) Check:

**Set**: Not a setting- it's measured from the ventilator.
**Check**: Pplat
**PIP > 30 cmHg**: Immediately switch to pressure control ventilation.

Plateau pressure is an indicator of alveolar pressures, and high Pplats indicate lung injury. Once a high Pplat is identified, you should transition your patient to pressure control ventilation immediately. It is important to transition to pressure control because it allows you to completely control the pressure that the lungs experience. If the lungs are repeatedly exposed to high pressures (> 30 cmH2O of Pplat) they will become damaged and pressure control prevents this.

Once all five of these finding are assessed, you can assume that you have patient-ventilator synchrony. At this point you will not notice any alarms (most likely) because the patient is synchronized to the ventilator. With the patient and ventilator synchronized, there will be much fewer alarms that sound because you have preemptively prevented the causes of these alarms. From this point, any alarm that sounds most likely will be something real and not frivolous.

### PRACTICE SESSION #18:

1. A high pressure alarm sounds and you not a PIP of 57 and a pPlat of 48? What is the significance of these findings?

2. The monitored data on the ventilator reads PIP 32 and pPlat of 29. What is the significance of these findings?
3. A high pressure alarm sounds and you not a PIP of 54 and a pPlat of 22? What is the significance of these findings?

SURFING EtCO2 and SpO2

Once you have ensured the patient's blood pressure is perfusing to the distal tissues, applied ventilator settings and minute ventilation that accommodate the patient's pH status, and double checked to make sure settings are fully reaching the patient's lungs, then you can begin making changes to the settings based on SpO2 and EtCO2. I call this "vent surfing" because you will read these vital signs and adjust the ventilator, just like you would read a wave and change directions when surfing. The conditions could be clam and constant, or it could be turbulent and consistently changing.

EtCO2

Remember that our EtCO2 status is incredibly reflective of our pH status. These two parameters are so closely connected that the literature agrees that we can use EtCO2 to make clinical decisions which would normally require pH data. The oxyhemoglobin dissociation curve suggests a low EtCO2 will cause hemoglobin to grasp oxygen tightly and not release it as it passes through the tissues. The oxyhemoglobin dissociation curve also suggests that a high EtCO2 causes hemoglobin to grasp oxygen very loosely, indicating that little oxygen gets attached to a red blood cell (RBC) for transport to the tissues. Both of these situations cause hypoxia by creating conditions that are not optimal for the on-load and off-load of oxygen onto the RBC. By utilizing the mechanical ventilator to target a normal EtCO2 (35-45 mmHg), we can optimize oxygen loading onto the RBC in the lung, as well as off-loading oxygen from the RBCs in the tissues.

Minute ventilation is the primary tool used to normalize EtCO2. If your patient has a high EtCO2, then you need a bigger 'shovel' to clear that acid therefore increase your minute ventilation. This can be achieved by increasing either RR, Vt, or PC. Since, RR x Vt = VE, increasing the respiratory rate (RR) or tidal volume (Vt) would elevate the minute ventilation thus reducing the EtCO2. Increasing the pressure control would also reduce the minute ventilation. Recall that pressure control (PC) is a setting on the ventilator when in pressure control ventilation. A normal initial PC is between 18- 22 ccH2O. A PC setting will deliver a narrow range of exhaled tidal volumes (Vte), nonetheless, if you increase a PC setting you are also increasing the tidal volume (or specifically Vte) the patient is experiencing. By this logic, if your EtCO2 is high, you could reduce it by raising the PC setting (if you are in pressure control mode). Reducing EtCO2 would simply work in the opposite direction: reducing RR, Vt, or PC will increase the EtCO2.

---

**VH Rule #12**: Correct EtCO2 by increasing or decreasing the RR, Vt, or the PC settings. These are directly proportional (↑ RR = ↑ minute ventilation).

---

SpO2

To prevent acidosis at the cellular level, we must collect and deliver oxygen to the tissues. Without oxygen at the tissues, the cells undergo anaerobic metabolism, creating acid as a byproduct. It is therefore paramount that we as clinicians ensure there is enough oxygen present so that the patient's metabolism remains aerobic enough to prevent acidosis.

To improve oxygenation, it is even simpler than correcting EtCO2. To increase a low SpO2, you would need to increase either the FiO2 or the PEEP. If your patient's SpO2 was 88%, by maximizing the FiO2 to 1.0 (or 100% oxygen delivery) you should see an increase in SpO2. Additionally, by increasing the PEEP you should see an improving SpO2.

---

**VH Rule #13**: Correct SpO2 by increasing the FiO2 or PEEP.

---

## PRACTICE SESSION #19:

1. Your patient has the following ventilator findings: RR 16, Vt 575, I:E 1:2, VE 9.1, SpO2 92, EtCO2 48, Pplat 17, Vte 572, and AutoPEEP 0. What changes to the ventilator can be made to correct the abnormal values?
2. Your patient has the following ventilator findings: RR vent assisted at 16 or 18, SpO2 98%, EtCO2 is 51, VE 8.9, f 18, Vte 556, PIP 17, Pplat 13, and AutoPEEP 0. What changes to the ventilator can be made to correct the abnormal values?

---

**The Universal Ventilator Approach (4 Step Process):**

1. **Ensure perfusion**
2. **Obtain Acid Status.**
3. **Choose vent settings and synchronize patient and vent.**
4. **Vent surf to obtain normal ranges of EtCO2 and SpO2.**

---

SUMMARY

The transport mechanical ventilator can be a scary piece of equipment if you do not practice it. However, if you realize that setting up a ventilator is as simple as ensuring a perfusing blood pressure, targeting minute volume, double checking to making sure that your settings are reaching the patient, and then simply make changes based on EtCO2 and SpO2 measurements, then this becomes a very attainable skill. The key is *practice, practice, practice*. Be sure to practice this skill over and over again. Practice by considering how you would set up a ventilator on every single patient, regardless of whether they actually need mechanical ventilation or not.

# 5 ADVANCED CONCEPTS

## EtCO2 AND SERUM CHANGES

I am confronted routinely with the concern that increasing a low EtCO2 in a patient with a low pH can be dangerous, and this is correct. A patient with metabolic acidosis will present with a low pH and a low EtCO2 or pCO2. What makes this particularly dangerous is the concurrent change in pH as EtCO2 (or pCO2) is elevated. You see, for every 10 mmHg in pCO2, there is an opposite change in pH by a factor of 0.1. Otherwise said, if you increase EtCO2 from 30 mmHg to 40 mmHg, then you should expect a DROP in pH by 0.1. This means that if you follow my suggestions of keeping the EtCO2 between 35-45 mmHg in a severe metabolic acidosis patient (who will present with low pH and low EtCO2) you could be harming the patient. Severe metabolic acidosis (defined by a low pH and a low pCO2) is a special situation where the EtCO2 or pCO2 should be maintained and not elevated. If the minute ventilation was reduced allowing the EtCO2 to elevate, the pH would drop even further in an acidotic patient.

Therefore, it is important to identify whether metabolic acidosis (indicated by a low pH and a low pCO2) is present before increasing a low EtCO2. An additional positive finding is the presence of an anion gap metabolic acidosis. By adding up the cations in the serum (Na and

K), and then subtracting the sum of all the anions of the serum (Cl and HCO3), we arrive at the anion gap. If this value is > 16, then an anion gap metabolic acidosis is present. This can help tip you off that metabolic acidosis is present.

Once a metabolic acidosis is identified, a savvy clinician will calculate the corrected $pCO_2$. This calculation can be made by the **Winter's formula**:

$$[pCO_2 = (1.5 \times HCO_3) + (8 +/- 2)].$$

Consider the following ABG: pH 7.10, $pCO_2$ 33, and HCO3 11. The pH and the $pCO_2$ are both low, therefore suggestive of metabolic acidosis. Apply the formula for $pCO_2$ correction and you get $pCO_2$ = $(1.5 \times 11) + (8) = 24 +/- 2$. Therefore, if you looked at this patient and tried to correct the low $EtCO_2$ by reducing minute ventilation, you would also be causing a more acidotic system.

---

**VH Rule #14**: In patients with low pH and low pCO2/ EtCO2, prevent further worsening acidosis by not elevating the low pCO2/ EtCO2.

---

The other side of the $pCO_2$ coin affects potassium. If you elevate $pCO_2$ by 10 mmHg, then you also elevate the potassium by 0.5 mEq/L. Therefore, in hyperkalemic patients, be careful about dropping the minute ventilation too low since that would drive up the $EtCO_2$ along with the potassium which would worsen the hyperkalemia.

**PRACTICE SESSION #20:**

1.    You patient has an $EtCO_2$ of 28 mmHg and a pH of 7.24. Why would reducing minute ventilation in this case be dangerous?
2.    Using Winter's formula, calculate the corrected $pCO_2$ from the following data: pH 7.25, $pCO_2$ 30, HCO3 12, $pO_2$ 99, BE -1.

## INITIATION VS. MAINTENANCE

You could subdivide your ventilator management experiences into two basic categories: 1) initiating the ventilator (starting from scratch), and 2)maintaining mechanical ventilation (patient already on vent and you just need to make changes). You will respond to hundreds of calls in your career when the patient will require mechanical ventilation. One type of call occurs where the patient is already receiving mechanical ventilation and your job is to determine if the settings are adequate. The second type of call involves initiating mechanical ventilation. The first is the easier of the two simply because there is less work to do.

It is important to cultivate a systematic approach when assessing either of these types of calls. For the first type of call (mechanical ventilation already established) you need to first assess SpO2. If the reading isn't 95% or higher than you need to increase either the FiO2 or the PEEP to correct the low SpO2. Next, track your eyes to the EtCO2 reading. If it is abnormal then you adjust the rate or tidal volume. If your patient is receiving pressure control ventilation, then you'll, of course, need to change the tidal volume by increasing or decreasing the pressure control setting. From this point you simply "vent surf"- adjust vital sign specific settings (Vt, RR, or PC for EtCO2; FiO2 and PEEP for SpO2).

For the second type of call you will need execute the full 4 step universal ventilator approach(page 71). As a review, ensure the blood pressure is perfusing the distal tissues. This ensures you'll be able to trust the vital signs SpO2 and EtCO2 which you'll use to make ventilator changes. Second, you will need to assess the patient's current pH status. This can be answered by asking three questions that indicates actual to potential acidosis. The questions are 1) is the pH low? (indicates actual acidosis), 2) is the patient breathing greater than 10 over their normal range? (strongly suggests an acidotic condition), and 3) is there an elevated EtCO2? (which potentially suggests an acidotic status- but is just a suggestion). If any of these questions are answered 'yes' then choose a target minute ventilation just outside the normal range for the patient. For an adult, 4-8 L/min minute ventilation is normal, so a 9 L/min on any acidotic patient would be a reasonable starting point. Thirdly, the clinician would need to calculate ideal body weight, tidal volume, and respiratory rate based on the chosen minute ventilation. Then set your non-calculated settings and ensure that your settings are reaching the patient. Once you achieve this, then the patient and the ventilator will be synchronized. Finally, you simply 'vent surf' by adjusting vital sign specific settings (Vt, RR, or PC for EtCO2; FiO2 and PEEP for SpO2).

## RECRUITMENT AND CLAMPING THE ET TUBE

There will be times you arrive at the patient's bedside to find an RT or physician who is incredibly protective of all the lung recruitment they have achieved. In ARDS patients, or any patient with inflamed and infected lungs, their lungs can develop atelectasis, also called alveolar collapse. When the lungs are infected or inflamed, they become very sticky and do not easily inflate. During an inspiration and as the difficulty to inflate the alveoli (from stickiness) is overcome, it aggravates the alveolar tissue. Think of Velcro. You really have to put in significant force to release Velcro, and that is the same problem with infected or inflamed lungs. Once the alveolar tissue is aggravated further inflammation and swelling occur. If this occurs enough, ARDS will develop. When this occurs, it may take clinicians hours to recruit lung volume enough to obtain adequate SpO2 and EtCO2 values. Recruiting lung volumes involves higher PEEPs to be able to splint open the alveoli thereby preventing collapse and the need to re-inflate as well as further alveolar aggravation. Once these clinicians achieve lung recruitment, they will be upset if you show up, remove them from the ventilator, and allow the lungs to collapse.

Typically recruitment occurs by maintaining a column of gas with higher PEEPs applied so that the alveoli do not have a chance to collapse. When lungs are inflamed or infected, this process could take hours as 1-2% of lung is recruited (re-inflated) with each passing minute. However, beware: if a clinician should remove this supporting column of gas by disconnecting the ventilator circuit from the patient's endotracheal tube, the recruitment is IMMEDIATELY lost and you'll have to start all over at a potential rate of 1-2% recruitment per minute. Do the math- this would take a while.

To prevent a loss of alveolar recruitment during transport, be prepared to clamp the endotracheal tube with hemostats. I understand this sounds crazy to some of you, but hold on to your chimichangas and I'll explain. To effectively perform this procedure and prevent a loss in recruitment, you will need to follow the following steps:

1.  Input your chosen settings into your transport ventilator and place the ventilator close to the patient.
2.  Using a test lung, or glove, begin cycling your ventilator.
3.  As the patient's ventilator is at maximum inspiration (noted by chest rise in your patient), clamp the patient's endotracheal tube with hemostats and gauze.
4.  Remove the patient from their ventilator and connect your transport ventilator to their endotracheal tube.
5.  As your transport ventilator is trying to deliver an inspiration against the clamped endotracheal tube, unclamp the tube as your transport ventilator is alarming "high pressure."

The ultimate goal in utilizing this procedure is to prevent any loss in alveolar recruitment, thereby creating more work for yourself and negating a lot of work that previous clinicians have put into improving the patient. The two key stages in this procedure are 1) clamping the endotracheal tube as the patient's ventilator is at maximum inspiration and 2) unclamping the endotracheal tube when the transport ventilator is trying to deliver a breath against the clamped endotracheal tube (thus causing a "high pressure" alarm). By ensuring these two components occur as described will guarantee a pressurized column of gas is always applied to the patient's pulmonary system which will minimize any loss of recruitment. **Additionally, be sure to use gauze when clamping to prevent cutting the endotracheal tube.**

Lastly, always be ready with a bougie and a replacement endotracheal tube should the hemostats cut the endotracheal tube. This highlights the importance of wrapping the endotracheal tube with a gauze at the clamp site. **The last thing you need is to be the idiot who just cut the patient's endotracheal tube. Conversely, completing this maneuver successfully literally makes you look like a rock star to most ICU personnel.**

## PRACTICE SESSION #21:

1.   Why is it important to unclamp the endotracheal tube when your transport ventilator is attempting to deliver positive breaths?
2.   You are about to clamp a patient's endotracheal tube for the first time and want to be prepared for any complications. What are some complications that can occur with this procedure?

## NON-INVASIVE POSITIVE PRESSURE VENTILATION

As you are becoming aware, the ventilator is an incredible machine. We have covered many of the invasive functions of the ventilator, but most transport ventilators have the capabilities of non-invasive procedures as well. What is intriguing is too often I'll engage in a conversation with a seasoned clinician about non-invasive positive pressure ventilation (NPPV), and they do not know when to choose bi-level positive airway pressure (BPAP) versus continuous positive airway pressure (CPAP). This section will discuss the finer points of NPPV.

It is important to keep in mind the main principles we have already addressed: correct $SpO2$ with PEEP and $FiO2$, and correct $EtCO2$ with RR and tidal volume (directly or with pressure control). These principles can be employed with invasive mechanical ventilation (meaning an endotracheal tube is in place) or with non-invasive positive pressure ventilation.

Consider an intubated patient on the mechanical ventilator who has a current $EtCO2$ of 51 mmHg and a $SpO2$ of 89%. To correct these two vital signs, we need to increase minute ventilation (to correct $EtCO2$) and increase $FiO2$ or $SpO2$ (to correct $SpO2$). This is, beautifully, the same methodology you execute when applying NPPV. Now, consider a CHF patient with the same vitals ($EtCO2$ of 51 mmHg and a $SpO2$ of 89%) who is awake. Using the same logic, a clinician could apply NPPV to an awake patient and still target lowering the $EtCO2$ and increasing the $SpO2$.

The problem most clinicians face is simply knowing when to apply CPAP and when to apply BPAP. To determine which mode is most appropriate for your patient, simply assess the patient's EtCO2 and SpO2. If the patient has a normal EtCO2 but a low SpO2, then the patient only needs oxygenation corrected, therefore CPAP is the appropriate setting. If the patient's SpO2 is low and the EtCO2 is abnormal, the patient needs both the oxygenation component as well as the ventilation component therefore BPAP is indicated. BPAP addresses both components, and therefore should be utilized anytime both SpO2 (oxygenation) and EtCO2 (ventilation) are abnormal.

---

**VH Rule #15**: In non-invasive positive pressure ventilation, use **CPAP** for oxygenation deficiencies and **BPAP** for oxygenation and ventilation deficiencies.

---

To set CPAP, you need to choose an expiratory positive airway pressure (EPAP). Interestingly, CPAP is essentially PEEP, therefore, the EPAP is also PEEP. Each of these three settings (CPAP, EPAP, and PEEP) all describe a constant pressure applied to a patient following the expiratory phase of a mechanically ventilated breath. It can be confusing, but take away from this the fact that these are all the same mechanism. The physiological benefit to these settings is the increase in surface area of alveoli and the thinning of the alveolar capillary membrane. These two actions increase the amount of oxygen that is diffused into the blood. A good starting point is the upper end of our normal physiologic PEEP, so 5 cmH2O. If more oxygenation is needed, then the EPAP (PEEP) setting needs to be increased. Some transport ventilators will allow you to change the EPAP setting or the PEEP setting, just remember that these are one in the same.

To improve ventilation in a patient with a high EtCO2, you can apply BPAP. To accomplish this, you would first set an inspiratory positive airway pressure (IPAP) and then you would set an EPAP. Therefore, you are setting a PEEP to remain following the expiratory phase, and also pressure support during the inspiratory phase.

Please keep in mind the mechanism of what we are doing, because some ventilators approach setting these pressures differently and you'll need to be able to discern the difference. Ultimately what we are doing in BPAP is setting a PEEP and a pressure support (PS) in an awake patient. They will control the RR, and we control the pressures. Remember that we cannot apply PS in assist control mode because each patient breath is fully assisted with the pre-set tidal volume or pressure control? It's possible in SIMV because the patient is allowed, occasionally, to take a breath on their own power- just like when they are awake on NPPV! So, for BPAP we set a PEEP (5 is a good starting point) and then we set a PS (10-15 are good starting points). If we want to utilize CPAP alone, then we simply set PEEP at 5 cmH2O, the RR to zero, and coach the patient to breathe in a comfortable manner.

Most transport ventilators allow you to set the IPAP, and then adds the IPAP and the EPAP (or PEEP) to get the peak inspiratory pressure, or the highest possible pressure. Therefore, the EPAP (or PEEP) is the lowest pressure in the airway while the PIP is the highest. The difference in the highest pressure (PIP) and the lowest pressure (EPAP, PEEP) is a pressure called the Delta-P. The Delta-P is derived from subtracting the EPAP from the PIP and ultimately represents the IPAP. So, if IPAP + EPAP = PIP, then IPAP = PIP – EPAP.

Some of you might be doubting this, so let me clarify. The debate we are having involves the concepts of additive pressure versus absolute pressures. Additive pressures are typically seen in hospital and transport ventilators where the PS is added to the PEEP to arrive at the expected PIP. Some transport ventilators and standalone (home) machines use absolute pressures which they confusingly term IPAP and EPAP. I know this is confusing, so I will tag the absolute terms with an asterisk to keep this at least a little less confusing. Now, in absolute versions of NPPV, the IPAP* is set and represents the PIP as it is the highest pressure. Then the EPAP* is set and represents PEEP. Therefore, PS is set based on the difference in IPAP* and EPAP*. Keep in mind, even in this case, there is still pressure support applied and a PEEP applied, but it is communicated differently using the terms IPAP* and EPAP*. The absolute pressures are delivered by home BPAP and CPAP machines as well as some transport ventilators. Be sure to know how your transport ventilator operates in this capacity.

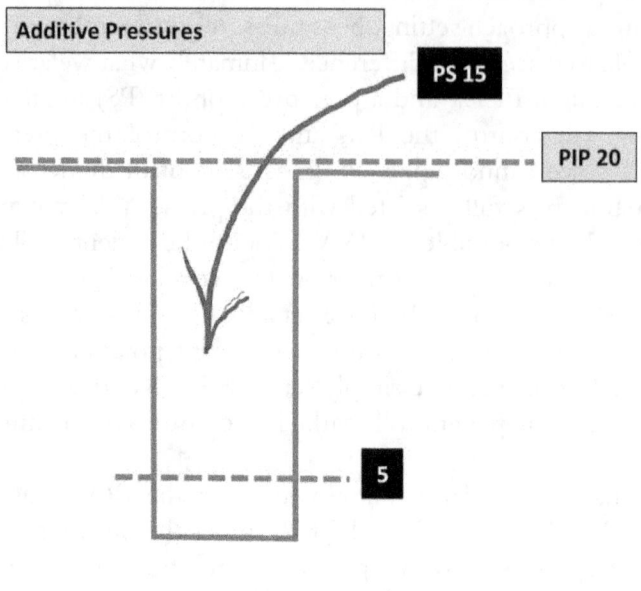

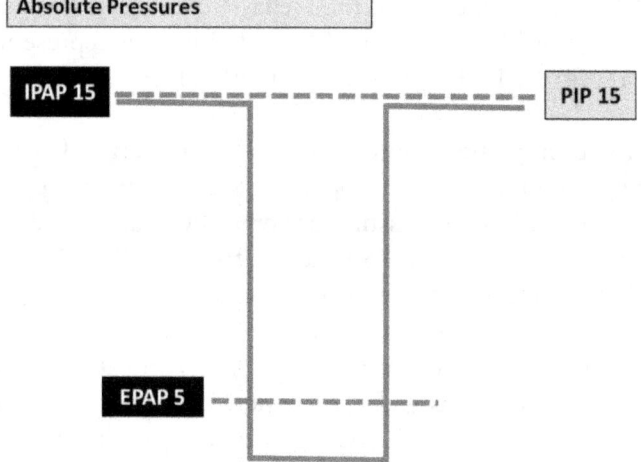

Be sure to test out this logic at your base to determine if your ventilator is additive or absolute. There usually are two methods to enter into NPPV mode of ventilation: through the front door and the back door. The 'front door' method is began by simply choosing the "NPPV" mode. It will ask to set an IPAP. Choose 15 cmH2O. Then it will ask you to set EPAP. Choose 5 cmH2O and have the ventilator begin. You'll have to simulate a patient's breath by gently squeezing the test lung, and then the 'patient' will be provided with a PS breath. Assess the PIP on the ventilator. If the PIP is 20 cmH2O, then your machine is additive (because the IPAP 15 + EPAP 5 = PIP 20). If the PIP is 15 cmH2O, then your ventilator is absolute (because the IPAP is 15 and therefore the PIP is 15).

The second method to enter into NPPV, is to select SIMV and turn the RR to zero. You'll need to set the SIMV mode which gives you the option of providing BPAP (remember, SIMV is needed to allow patient to breath under their own power). If you want to deliver BPAP, then set the PS to 10 or 15 cmH2O and then set the PEEP to 5. If you want to set CPAP, then turn the PS down to zero and the PEEP to 5 cmH2O. Yes, it is that simple. I prefer this method because I am not confused if the "IPAP" is precalculating the PIP (absolute) or if it is giving me the 2 different pressures of PS and PEEP (additive). In this way, you always know that the PEEP you set is being delivered in tandem with the set pressure support (in BPAP mode). It simply makes it less confusing.

To make changes with CPAP or BPAP, simply use the principles we have already drilled into your heads. If your patient has a SpO2 of 90, then increase PEEP or FiO2. BE CAREFUL WITH INCREASING FiO2- this can drain down your oxygen tank (see next section). Keep the FiO2 as minimumal as possible. If your EtCO2 is high, simply increase the PS setting, but make sure you communicate this change to your patient. They may get spooked by the smallest change, so just keep them informed.

### Common Initial Settings:
1. IPAP: 10-15 cmH2O
2. EPAP: 5-10 cmH2O

**Note: the larger the IPAP and EPAP difference, the greater effect on minute ventilation.**

## PRACTICE SESSION #22:

1. You have a patient with CHF and you decide to attempt non-invasive positive pressure ventilation. Currently, the patient has these findings: HR 102, RR 24, SpO2 85, and EtCO2 41. Which type of NPPV is warranted here?
2. Your COPD patient is short of breath and has the following findings: HR 82, RR 18, SpO2 88, and EtCO2 61. Which type of NPPV is warranted here?


OXYGEN CALCULATIONS

In today's medical transport world, especially in the aviation realm, calculating oxygen can be difficult because of the various different types of oxygen tank materials, different pressurizations, differing volumes, and unclear sources to use to calculate your oxygen tank durations. In the past, all you had to do was to memorize a tank factor that was well utilized and tested, like a D tank. The D tank is the common portable O2 tank size that has been widely used for decades. The tank factor is 0.16, so, by multiplying this factor by the current pressure in the tank, you arrive at the total available liters of oxygen in the tank. Then you divide that result by the liter flow (L/min) of the oxygen delivery device to arrive at your duration (in minutes) of oxygen.

The problem you'll find, or likely have already found, today is that there is a new universe of oxygen tanks and cylinders now making it daunting to identify the correct tank factor, let alone try to calculate one. Luckily, there is a simple formula to derive the tank factor for any oxygen tank. The tank factor, also called 'cal factor', is the total liters of oxygen gas divided by the max pressure of the tank containing the oxygen (total L O2/ tank PSI). It's that simple.


**Oxygen Tank Cal Factor Formula = (Total liters of O2)/(max oxygen tank fill pressure)**

The difficulty usually comes with obtaining the total liters of oxygen in a tank, also called tank capacity. Oxygen volume can be described in a tank as cubic feet, cubic inches, or (ideally) in liters. Some manufacturers prefer using cubic feet or cubic liters therefore, forcing one more calculation upon us. To convert cubic feet to liters, multiply the given cubic feet by 28.33, and the result is the number of liters (L) in the container. To convert cubic inches to liters, multiply the given cubic inches by 0.016, and the result is the number of liters (L) in the container. You can obtain tank information from your oxygen provider or distributor. Additionally, you can go online to your oxygen provider's website. These oxygen companies typically have tank information easily accessible on their websites. Finally, most tanks will have capacity information on the tank itself, although not all states require this information. So, if you are in a state not requiring a company to put capacity information onto the tank in addition to using an oxygen provider who fails to put capacity information on the tank, then you will need to refer to the oxygen provider company's reference material. You should reach out immediately if you do not have this information on hand, and definitely before your next call or flight.

Once you know your tanks' maximum capacity and its maximum fill pressure then you're ready to calculate your tanks specific 'cal' factor. If you cannot find a maximum pressure, then you can look at the pressure gauge for several tanks that have not been used previously. Record the most commonly observed initial pressure that the company sends you, which can be seen once a tank is first opened. This pressure can substituted as the 'max pressure' and is more accurate that blindly calculating the tank's reported absolute max pressure. Most of the time an oxygen company will under-fill the tank relative to its maximum pressure. Due to this, using their common fill pressure would make your calculations more accurate.

Now that you have calculated your oxygen tanks cal factor, you can use it to calculate the duration of oxygen = [(cal factor x current PSI)/(flow rate of oxygen delivery device)]. This equation gives you time (in minutes) remaining in your oxygen tank at your current rate of oxygen delivery.

**Oxygen Cylinder Tank Duration Formula = [(cal factor) x (current PSI)/ oxygen flow rate)]**

Liquid Oxygen Systems

Oxygen can be efficiently stored if kept in its liquid form. Liquid oxygen, or LOX, is a very efficient method to carry lots of oxygen. Liquid oxygen is commonly seen in the medical aviation environment, so it is important to mention in this text.

Oxygen has an expansion ratio of 1:860, meaning that 1 L of liquid oxygen is equivalent to 860 L of gaseous oxygen. To calculate the duration of liquid oxygen, obtain the liters of liquid oxygen available in the tank by observing the liquid oxygen display panel in the aircraft. Once you have the liquid liters, you multiply it by 860. This results in the total number of gaseous liters of oxygen available. Next, you divide the total liters of gaseous oxygen by the current oxygen delivery flow rate (4 L/min nasal cannula or 15 L/min non-rebreather mask as an example) which results in the oxygen duration in minutes.

**LOX Tank Duration Formula = [(# liters of LOX x 860)/ oxygen flow rate)]**

Oxygen Delivery Devices

There are some common oxygen delivery devices that you're likely familiar with, such as nasal cannula or non-rebreather mask. These oxygen delivery devices have a range of flow rates. For instance, the nasal cannula has a flow rate range of 2-6 L/min and the non-rebreather mask has a flow rate range of 10-15 L/min. When retrieving a patient, simply note the current flow rate and plug it into a oxygen duration formula. What is difficult is using a CPAP/ BPAP machine or a mechanical ventilator because the flow rates with these devices can wax and wane. You can estimate the oxygen consumption by using some of these calculations below, but it is always best to routinely recalculate your oxygen duration every 20 minutes or so, and especially after every flow rate change.

To calculate the oxygen duration for a patient on a mechanical ventilator, you must take into account their minute ventilation, FiO2, the tank-specific cal factor, and the current PSI. So basically, you need to calculate oxygen just as we have discussed, but factor in how much air they are moving (minute ventilation) and how much of that is oxygen (FiO2). By completing this calculation, you have an estimate for the duration of your oxygen with a patient receiving mechanical ventilation at your chosen tidal volume and FiO2.

## Ventilator O2 Flow Formula = [(exhaled tidal volume)(respiratory rate)(FiO2)]

Where do you obtain the information to calculate this? You obtain it from the ventilator itself. It does not matter if you are ventilating the patient in invasive or non-invasive mode, you still obtain the same variables. First, you need to identify the minute ventilation, so you need to obtain the tidal volume. If the patient is receiving invasive mechanical ventilation (ventilation via an endotracheal tube) then you obtain the Vte from the ventilator and multiply it by the number of inspirations (frequency, $f$). Even if you are in pressure control mode, Vte multiplied by the frequency will provide the most accurate minute ventilation. Even simpler, you could obtain the minute ventilation form the monitored data panel on the vent. If your patient is receiving non- invasive positive pressure ventilation, you would calculate the minute ventilation by multiplying the patient's own respiratory rate by their Vte which you would obtain from the ventilator's monitored data panel.

Once you obtain the minute ventilation of your patient on the ventilator, you simply multiply this value by the FiO2. The result is the mechanical ventilator's flow rate which can be used for the basic equations we have already discussed. The caveat to this simplistic approach is <u>be careful</u>- there can be other forces not easily calculated acting on oxygen consumption, so be careful not to run out of oxygen because of a unidentified leak. As a ventilator conducts its medical business, oxygen can leak and equipment flow can be more than what is calculated. **The transport mechanical ventilator is a fickle, fickle** apparatus, and as such O2 consumption will never be exactly as calculated. Therefore, we need to constantly re-calculate our oxygen consumption to reaffirm the amount and duration. Just like a patient's blood pressure, it could decompensate at any time, so we need to re-evaluate often to ensure we have enough O2 reserve to complete the flight, call, or mission.

# Formulas:

**Oxygen Tank Cal Factor Formula** = (Total liters of O2)/(max oxygen tank fill pressure)

**Oxygen Cylinder Tank Duration Formula** = [(cal factor x current PSI)/ oxygen flow rate)]

**LOX Tank Duration Formula** = [(# liters of LOX x 860)/ oxygen flow rate)]

**Ventilator O2 Flow Formula** = [(exhaled tidal volume)(respiratory rate)(FiO2)]

## PRACTICE SESSION #23:

1. You have an oxygen tank that is 660 L in capacity and has a max fill pressure of 1900 PSI. What is the cal factor for this oxygen tank?
2. Your ventilated patient has a minute ventilation of 6 L/min and an FiO2 of 0.7. What is this patient's ventilator cal factor?
3. You have an oxygen tank that is 500 L in capacity and has a max fill pressure of 2100 PSI. Your ventilated patient has a minute ventilation of 9 L/min and an FiO2 of 0.9. What is the duration of your oxygen tank?

# MANEUVERS AS DIAGNOSTICS

In chapter 1 we discussed the maneuvers functions. There are two: the inspiratory hold maneuver and the expiratory hold maneuver. As a review, the inspiratory hold maneuver provides us with the plateau pressure and the expiratory hold provides us with the AutoPEEP. The plateau pressure indicates the elasticity and healthiness of the lung and AutoPEEP tells us if breath stacking is occurring. A healthy and elastic lung presents with a plateau pressure less than 30 cmH2O. Plateau pressures higher than this 30 cmH2O threshold damages lung tissue. Additionally, as long as breaths are not conducted too fast to prevent alveolar and airway emptying, then the AutoPEEP should be < 0. If we breathe too fast, then we begin autoPEEPing, or also known as breath- stacking.

Inspiratory Hold Maneuver

If we were working a shift together and I ask you to put a patient on 1200 cc of tidal volume, you most likely would question me about which setting. Chances are you'd at least ask if I was sure about such a large tidal volume. Think about why it concerns you. In medicine, when we learn to administer a therapy, we learn when to administer it (indications), we learn when not to administer it (contraindications), and we learn what happens when too much is given (toxicology). The ventilator should be approached with the same methodology, but too often the toxic elements are not well understood. Consider the 1200 cc applied to a hypothetical patient. Is this a toxic dose? Will it hurt an adult patient? A pediatric? An infant? Your gut may say 'yes' but can you explain it?

Any volume can potentially injure a patient. We tend to think of 'dangerous tidal volumes' as the upper end of a normal range someone insisted you us memorize from a textbook. However, a dangerous tidal volume is one that generates a plateau pressure greater than 30 cmH2O. Therefore, monitoring plateau pressures becomes diagnostic in predicting the safety or danger in administering high tidal volumes. Bottom line: if your Pplat is < 30 cmH2O, you <u>are not</u> damaging lung tissue.

The literature corroborates this concept and adds that PEEP also plays a role in preventing lung injury. Atelectasis is the de-recruitment (or deflation) of the alveoli during exhalation. If alveoli are allowed to completely, or near completely; deflate, then lung injury can occur as the sticky and inflamed deflated alveolar walls touch one another during exhalation. Because they are sticky, these collapsed walls adhere to one another. During the next inspiratory cycle, an inspiratory breath forcefully separates them (like in the Velcro analogy from earlier). This forceful separation can cause microtrauma which leads to the activation of the inflammatory system. What happens if the inflammatory system is turned loose in the alveolar system? That's right- ARDS occurs. Therefore, we maintain PEEP in our mechanically ventilated patients to help prevent the damage of lung tissue.

The bottom line in this case is centered around plateau pressure and PEEP. Plateau pressure becomes a diagnostic indicator of lung injury. If we maintain PEEP and routinely check plateau pressure, then lung injury can be prevented. You can deliver high tidal volumes safely (yes, even 1000, 1200, or more cc of tidal volume) as long as your plateau pressure is lower than 30 cmH2O. Utilize the inspiratory hold maneuver (volume control mode only) to accomplish obtaining routine plateau pressures.

Expiratory Hold Maneuver

What would the danger be in applying a respiratory rate too high? Just like in the tidal volume discussion, avoid selecting an answer that is based on a "normal range". True, normal range is important, but the question isn't 'what is normal', the question is 'what is dangerous.' To answer this, consider the concern with breathing at too fast a rate. Eventually, we can breathe so fast that we progress to the inspiratory phase before the exhalation phase is completed. This causes breath stacking, or known on the mechanical ventilator as AutoPEEP.

AutoPEEP is a measured data point on mechanical ventilators that is measured in cmH2O over the preset PEEP setting. By executing the expiratory hold maneuver, a clinician can obtain the AutoPEEP value and therefore detect the presence of breath stacking. If AutoPEEP is recorded as "0" or "< 0", then no breath stacking is occurring and the current RR is not dangerous. If AutoPEEP is recorded as a positive number, then that number represents the extra PEEP that is occurring thus indicating the set RR is dangerously fast. It is possible to observe AutoPEEPs of 1 and 2, but at an AutoPEEP of 3 and above, most ventilators will alarm with the 'high PEEP' alarm.

If AutoPEEP is identified, simply increase the expiratory phase of the I:E ratio. This can be accomplished by turning down the I-time setting which in effect increases the E-time. This allows for a longer expiratory phase and can help reduce (or clear out) the AutoPEEP. Once you set an I:E ratio with a lover expiratory phase, reassess the AutoPEEP. If the reading is "< zero" then you're no longer AutoPEEPing. If the AutoPEEP is a positive whole number, then you are still AutoPEEPing, and need to repeat the procedure just mentioned to increase the I:E ratio to allow for a greater exhalation time.

In summary, the inspiratory hold and expiratory hold maneuvers can be used as diagnostics and help to identify if the RR or Vt are dangerously high. If you are ventilating in volume control ventilation and you want to monitor if your Vt is safe, obtain the plateau pressure data from an inspiratory hold maneuver. If you are in volume control ventilation and you want to identify if the preset RR is too high, momentarily switch to pressure control ventilation, execute an expiratory hold maneuver, and then switch back to volume control. If AutoPEEP is a positive number, then increase the expiratory phase of the I:E ratio by reducing the I-time, which in turn increases the E-time. In summary, the inspiratory hold maneuver and the expiratory hold maneuver provide diagnostic evidence as to the safety of the RR and Vt.

## PRACTICE SESSION #24:

1. You have set an I:E ratio for your patient who is having an asthmatic attack. How can you identify if this I:E ratio is appropriate?
2. Explain how we can change our treatment by utilizing the inspiratory hold maneuver.

# THE FLUIDITY OF MAKING VENTILATOR CHANGES

Keep in mind the ventilator is an incredibly dynamic piece of machinery, and when it is coupled with actual live tissue it becomes even more dynamic. In this section, we will discuss some expectations to particular ventilator changes to instill in you an awareness of how one change will affect a different setting, thus changing your vitals or monitored data. Being able to anticipate these changes will keep you in control and prevent confusion.

## I:E Ratio and Respiratory Rate

While the transport ventilator is an amazing piece of equipment, it isn't without flaws. One of these flaws in in the form of having to 'babysit' I:E ratio each time you change the respiratory rate. Most transport ventilators keep the I-time static, meaning it will not change as you make other ventilator changes. This means each time you change the respiratory rate, the I-time remains the same and the I:E ratio changes.

This can be explained with the following scenario: consider a patient on the ventilator set at a respiratory rate of 12. This means each breath lasts 5 seconds (or the total cycle time is 5 seconds). If the I-time is set at 1.0, then the calculation is easy. Inspiration is 1 second and expiration is composed of the remaining 4. This equates to an I:E ratio of 1:4. Now, suppose we increase this patient's respiratory rate to 20. This would mean that the total cycle time would now be 3 seconds. Recall the I-time remains static, so at 1.0 the inspiratory phase is now 1 second and the expiratory phase is 2 seconds. This equates to an I:E ratio of 1:2.

So you see, by changing the respiratory rate, you'll need to always follow it up with a change of I:E ratio. With the transport ventilator, I usually do not care too much about the I-time, although it does have a huge place in mechanical ventilation. What I typically suggest to make changes to the I:E ratio is to select the I-time button on the transport ventilator, cover up the I-time value, and change the setting while monitoring the actual calculated I:E ratio the ventilator displays in the monitored data panel. This way you will not get bogged down with trying to calculate E-times, total cycle times, and I:E ratios- it does it for you.

PEEP and Vte

Recall that PEEP is the leftover pressure in the lungs after exhalation and before the next inspiration. This means that any pressure (if in pressure control) or tidal volume (if in volume control) sent into the lung must be stacked onto this pressure. As you add more and more PEEP, you essentially leave the lung more and more filled. As you increase the PEEP, you can expect changes in both exhaled tidal volume (Vte) and minute ventilation (VE). Therefore, you should also see concomitant increases in EtCO2 since minute ventilation is decreasing. To combat this phenomenon, simply increase the Vt, PC, or RR to increase minute ventilation (like always). The RR may be more effective in this case because it is not associated with lung volume, which PEEP affects. Bottom line: monitor EtCO2 always and make appropriate changes to keep it in normal ranges.

The Fickle Ventilator and the Fall Back

Always keep in mind that the mechanical ventilator is a machine which is being applied to human tissue. It is an imperfect process and set of procedures. The data that we monitor to keep things in balance can change just like a patient's blood pressure or heart rate can change during a transport. We need to be ready to act, and sometimes act without truly understanding what happened. We can always fall back on guiding ventilator changes based on SpO2 and EtCO2. If Vte drops for an unknown reason, be sure to return minute ventilation back to normal by increasing the respiratory rate. If adding PEEP drops a patient's blood pressure, then administer fluids, blood, or pressors (depending on what is going on with the patient) to support the blood pressure.

## PRACTICE SESSION #25:

1.   Your patient is in ARDS and you have had to titrate up PEEP to 17 cmH2O to be able to oxygenate the patient. You notice a low minute ventilation alarm sounding. Explain why this alarm sounded.
2.   You change the RR on your patient and later notice that they are autoPEEPing. Explain why this happened.


## PRESSURE REGULATED VOLUME CONTROL

So you really want to know about PRVC? Well here's a spoiler: you already do. Your new found knowledge of pressure control is the key to understanding this ventilation mode.

Consider the following case: you have a patient that you decide to try out pressure control ventilation, so you set the pressure control at 20 cmH2O. Once the ventilator starts delivering breaths, you notice the exhaled tidal volume (Vte) is 850 cc. Prior to initiating the ventilator you calculated this patient required 550 cc. So, like an astute clinician of the ventilator, you dial down the pressure control setting to 15 cmH2O. You then receive feedback from the ventilator that the Vte is now 400 cc. Next, you increase the pressure control setting to 18 cmH2O. The ventilator now reads a Vte of 675 cc. After multiple attempts to identify the right pressure control setting to achieve your desired tidal volume, you find that 16 cmH2O results in Vte(s) close to 550 cc. If you understand and follow this line of changes, then you already know about PRVC.

PRVC is a dual mode of ventilation. This means that it marries the two major driving forces that are possible with the mechanical ventilator: pressure control ventilation and volume control ventilation. Recall that in volume control ventilation we set a particular tidal volume, and then monitor the pressures that volume creates. We are usually guaranteed a particular minute ventilation, which is a characteristic feature of volume control ventilation. As in the above scenario, pressure control ventilation is centered around choosing a particular pressure limit, which we call the pressure

94

control setting, and monitoring the volumes that reach the patient (Vte). If we detect the pressure control is delivering too high or too low of a tidal volume, then we adjust the pressure control setting lower or higher, respectively, to ensure a near constant minute ventilation. Pressure regulated volume control (PRVC) is a mode that harnesses the benefits of both pressure control ventilation and volume control ventilation.

PRVC works by setting a pressure control, monitoring the Vte from breath to breath, and then makes changes to the pressure control to ensure that the Vte matches the desired title volume. If you think back to the scenario that began this section, you will notice that the scenario played out exactly as PRVC operates: a desired tidal volume is set on the ventilator, a pressure control is chosen (by the ventilator's microprocessor), each breath is measured to ensure that the chosen pressure will deliver the desired tidal volume, and finally the ventilator will make automatic changes to the delivered pressure to ensure the desired tidal volume reaches the patient.

Ultimately, you already know how to utilize this mode. This is one of the first "smart modes" in the transport ventilator arsenal, and it is becoming increasingly popular. This is a very safe mode because it harnesses both the benefits of pressure control ventilation (more efficient breath delivery, maintaining lower airway pressures) as well as volume control ventilation (guaranteed minute ventilation). By blending some of the best features of each of these modes provides the clinician with a very safe dual mode of mechanical ventilation.

Setting PRVC:

1. Choose volume control ventilation
2. Choose PRVC
3. Set your tidal volume, respiratory rate, I: E ratio, PEEP, and FiO2.
4. Set pressure limit
5. Apply to patient.

# 6 THE 15 VENT HERO RULES

1. You can still aim for a specific minute volume in PRESSURE CONTROL ventilation.

2. If your patient is chemically paralyzed, or adequately sedated, then the mode you apply doesn't matter. Mode decides what the ventilator will do if they are awake to take a breath and it isn't our job in transport medicine is not to wean our patients from the ventilator.

3. With a transport ventilator, every time you readjust respiratory rate, then readjust the I:E ratio.

4. If PEEP earns you improved oxygenation but drops BP, do not remove PEEP! Instead support BP with fluids, blood and/or pressors.

5. Pressure support can only be applied in SIMV mode because it is the only mode where the patient has the ability to take a breath own power.

6. High PIP and normal pPlat = a resistance problem; high PIP and high pPlat = a compliance problem.

7. Never assume you can seamlessly replicate the settings from one ventilator to a transport ventilator- ever.

8. Low blood pressure gives provides unreliable EtCO2 and SpO2 values.

9. Stop guessing on minute ventilation. Start using the information the patient provides you.

10. Never assume your settings are reaching the vent. Prove to yourself the desired settings are reaching the patient.

11. If you fail to ensure that what you set is reaching the patient, then you ensure ventilator failure.

12. Correct SpO2 by increasing the FiO2 or PEEP.

13. Correct SpO2 by increasing the FiO2 or PEEP.

14. In non-invasive positive pressure ventilation, use CPAP for oxygenation deficiencies and biPAP for oxygenation and ventilation deficiencies.

15. In non-invasive positive pressure ventilation, use CPAP for oxygenation deficiencies and biPAP for oxygenation and ventilation deficiencies.

# 7 CASE STUDIES

In the following pages you will be presented with 10 different case studies designed to test your knowledge. The case studies are delivered in a 4 page format. The first page presents the case and has workspace to document blood pressure data; to calculate IBW, tidal volume, and respiratory rate based off a specifically chosen minute ventilation; to choose PEEP, FiO2, and I:E ratio; and finally to identify patient ventilator synchrony data. Follow the procedure of applying the universal ventilator strategy.

On the second case study page, an update will be provided. After the update, you will be prompted to consider if pain management, sedation, and/or paralytic medications are required. You will then be prompted to identify or correct high pressure issues, minute ventilation issues, and oxygenation issues. The third page provides a second update along with the same sedation, pain medication, paralysis, high pressure, ventilation, and oxygenation, just as on the second page. The fourth page is the rationale for all the previous pages and ultimately explains how to best treat the patients provided in the scenarios.

Use the following pages as a first test run for this knowledge and practice you have just read about. Too often we listen and understand, but fail to effectively practice. You be the catalyst to help ensure we as clinicians become much better at this enigma that is called the mechanical ventilator.

**Case# 1**

---

**INITIAL**: A patient with DKA has just been intubated for altered mental status. The patient weighs 195 lbs and is 6'1". His vital signs are HR 121, BP 135/86 with strong radial pulse, RR assisted at 22/min via BVM, SpO2 89%, and EtCO2 is 62.

---

**Step 1: BP:**    Absent/ Weak/ Present

    Corrective Action:

**Step 2: Acidosis**: Present/ Suspected/ Possible/ Absent

    Target VE: _____
        IBW: (2.3)(___ inches > 60 inches) + 50 or 45.5 = ___
        ITV: (6-8 cc)(IBW) = _____
        RR: VE _____ / ITV _____ = RR _____

        PEEP: _____
        I:E: _____
        FiO2: _____

**Step 3: Patient/ Ventilator Synchrony:**
Below are some possible settings and findings. If the provided values do not match, provide the corrective action.

    $VE_{EXPECTED}$ __9.4__ vs. $VE_{ACTUAL}$ __14.4__    Match?  Yes/ No

        Corrective Action:

    RR __17__ vs. f __26__    Match?  Yes/ No

        Corrective Action:

    Vt __560__ vs. Vte __550__    Match?  Yes/ No

        Corrective Action:

    PIP: __18__ Pplat: __13__    Under normal safe limits? Yes/ No

> **UPDATE 1**: ALARM: High minute ventilation. Your patient's vital signs and measured vent data are BP 126/82 with strong radial pulses, HR 122, RR vent assisted at 16 or 18, SpO2 91%, EtCO2 is 41, VE 14.4, Vt 560, f 26, Vte 555, PIP 18, Pplat 13, and AutoPEEP 0.

**Changes in sedation/ pain medication/ paralysis needed?** Yes/ No

If YES, explain why:

**High pressure an issue?** Yes/ No

If YES, can you r/o the DOPE acronym?

If you cannot r/o DOPE, did you switch to PC? Yes/ No

Rationale/ Notes:

**Do you need to correct minute ventilation?** Yes/ No

If so, which require changing? _____ RR/ ____TV/ ____PC

Rationale/ Notes:

**Do you need to correct the oxygenation?** Yes/ No

If so, which require correction? _____ FiO2/ _____ PEEP

Rationale/ Notes:

---

**UPDATE 2**: Minute ventilation has been corrected by sedating the patient and returning the frequency back to match the set RR. There is no alarm currently sounding. Current vent settings are volume control in A/C mode with RR 16 or 18, I:E 1:2, Vt 560, PEEP 5, and FiO2 of 1.0. Your patient's vital signs and measured vent data are BP 130/84 with strong radial pulses, HR 102, RR vent assisted at 16 or 18, SpO2 98%, EtCO2 is 51, VE 8.9, f 16 or 18, Vte 556, PIP 17, Pplat 13, and AutoPEEP 0.

---

**Changes in sedation/ pain medication/ paralysis needed?**  Yes/ No

> If YES, explain why:

**High pressure an issue?**  Yes/ No

> If YES, can you r/o the DOPE acronym?

> If you cannot r/o DOPE, did you switch to PC?  Yes/ No

> Rationale/ Notes:

**Do you need to correct minute ventilation?**  Yes/ No

> If so, which require changing?  _____ RR/ _____TV/ _____PC

> Rationale/ Notes:

**Do you need to correct the oxygenation?**  Yes/ No

> If so, which require correction?  _____ FiO2/ _____ PEEP

> Rationale/ Notes:

## Case #1: Explanation and Rationale

**General Impression**:

---

**Initial Rationale**:
BP: Adequate (appears adequate)
Acidosis: potentially present (high EtCO2)
Target VE: most likely- begin at 9L/min or 10 L/min
IBW: 79.9, or rounded to 80 kg
ITV: 560 (80 kg x 7 cc/kg of tidal volume)
RR: (target VE/ ITV=RR); 9000/560= RR 16 or 10000/ 560= 18
I:E 1:2 (no evidence of bronchospasm and patient isn't a pediatric)
FiO2: 1.0 (we are initiating, so start high and titrate down as quickly as the SpO2 allows)
PEEP: 5 cmH2O ( start at this upper end of normal)
Actions needed to sync: The f and VE are both high. Sedate the patient or increase vent sensitivity to return VE and f back to the desired ranges.

---

**UPDATE 1 Rationale:**
EtCO2: Normal.
SpO2: Still low, but improved. Continue to increase FiO2 or PEEP.
Alarms: high minute ventilation. Cause: increased frequency (f) of 26/min compared to the preset RR of 16 or 18. The f of 26 x Vte of 560 equals our measured VE of 14.4 L/min, and therefore strongly suggests the rationale of high minute ventilation due to high frequency most likely from the patient being under sedated. Also, a low sensitivity causes the vent to be triggered if vibrations are too high. Fix: 1) increase sensitivity setting and 2) sedate and/or paralyze the patient to prevent patient initiated attempts.

---

**UPDATE 2 Rationale**:
EtCO2: now high- most likely because the patient before was over breathing the vent and self-correcting. After you paralyze or sedate, the patient's f now matches the RR. This brings minute ventilation back closer to normal and to the initially calculated VE of 9 or 10 L/min. Fix: increase minute ventilation to about 14 L/min, which the patient was over-breathing to get an EtCO2 between normal ranges. Doing so brings the EtCO2 down to 43 mmHg.
SpO2: Corrected.
Alarms: no alarms.

---

**Case# 2**                                                    Date: _____

---

**INITIAL**: A trauma patient with chest trauma has just been intubated. The patient is a male who weighs 225 lbs and is 6'4". His vital signs are HR 112, BP 82/63 with no radial pulse, RR assisted at 20/min via BVM, SpO2 83%, and EtCO2 is 29.

---

**Step 1: BP:**    Absent/ Weak/ Present

Corrective Action:

**Step 2: Acidosis**: Present/ Suspected/ Possible/ Absent

Target VE: _____
    IBW: (2.3)(___ inches > 60 inches) + 50 or 45.5 = ___
    ITV: (6-8 cc)(IBW) = _____
    RR: VE _____ / ITV _____ = RR _____

PEEP: _____
    I:E: _____
    FiO2: _____

**Step 3: Patient/ Ventilator Synchrony:**
Below are some possible settings and findings. If the provided values do not match, provide the corrective action.

VE$_{EXPECTED}$ _7.8_ vs. VE$_{ACTUAL}$ _7.7_    Match?  Yes/ No

    Corrective Action:

RR _13_ vs. f _13_    Match?  Yes/ No

    Corrective Action:

Vt _610_ vs. Vte _605_    Match?  Yes/ No

    Corrective Action:

PIP: _21_ Pplat: _17_    Under normal safe limits? Yes/ No

> **UPDATE 1**: Your patient's vital signs and measured vent data are BP 104/78 with strong radial pulses, HR 102, RR 13, SpO2 98, EtCO2 51, PIP 21, Pplat 17, Vte 605, f 13, and AutoPEEP 0. Current vent settings are volume control in SIMV mode with RR 13, I:E 1:2, Vt 610, PEEP 5, and FiO2 of 1.0.

**Changes in sedation/ pain medication/ paralysis needed?** Yes/ No

   If YES, explain why:

**High pressure an issue?** Yes/ No

   If YES, can you r/o the DOPE acronym?

   If you cannot r/o DOPE, did you switch to PC? Yes/ No

   Rationale/ Notes:

**Do you need to correct minute ventilation?** Yes/ No

   If so, which require changing? _____ RR/ _____TV/ _____PC

   Rationale/ Notes:

**Do you need to correct the oxygenation?** Yes/ No

   If so, which require correction? _____ FiO2/ _____ PEEP

   Rationale/ Notes:

UPDATE 2: Current vent settings are volume control in SIMV mode with RR 17 (increased to elevate minute ventilation this lower EtCO2), I:E 1:2, Vt 610, PEEP 5, and FiO2 of 1.0. Your patient's vital signs and measured vent data are BP 130/84 with strong radial pulses, HR 102, SpO2 99%, EtCO2 is 47, VE 10.2, f 17, Vte 605, PIP 17, Pplat 13, and AutoPEEP 0.

**Changes in sedation/ pain medication/ paralysis needed?** Yes/ No

If YES, explain why:


**High pressure an issue?** Yes/ No

If YES, can you r/o the DOPE acronym?

If you cannot r/o DOPE, did you switch to PC? Yes/ No

Rationale/ Notes:


**Do you need to correct minute ventilation?** Yes/ No

If so, which require changing? _____ RR/ _____TV/ _____PC

Rationale/ Notes:


**Do you need to correct the oxygenation?** Yes/ No

If so, which require correction? _____ FiO2/ _____ PEEP

Rationale/ Notes:

## Case #2: Explanation and Rationale

### General Impression:

> **Initial Rationale:**
> BP: inadequate so admin fluids (500cc to 1L is a good starting point).
> Acidosis: not currently evident but be prepared to correct hypercapnia once perfusion is restored. A spike in EtCO2 occurs after a return of perfusion.
> Target VE: most likely- begin at 8 L/min or 9 L/min
> IBW: 86.8, or 87 kg
> ITV: 609 cc
> RR: (target VE/ ITV=RR); 8000/609= RR 13 or 9000/ 560= 15
> I:E 1:2 (no evidence of bronchospasm and patient isn't a pediatric)
> FiO2: 1.0 (we are initiating, so start high and titrate down as quickly as the SpO2 allows)
> PEEP: 5 cmH2O (start at this upper end of normal)
> Actions needed to sync: none needed. Settings and monitored data match pretty closely.

> **UPDATE 1 Rationale:**
> EtCO2: Now high- most likely from returning perfusion allowing excessive amounts of CO2 to be picked up at the tissues. Fix: increase minute ventilation (increase RR or Vt).
> SpO2: corrected.
> Alarms: none.

> **UPDATE 2 Rationale:**
> EtCO2: still high- but improving. Fix: Keep increasing minute ventilation- increase minute ventilation to about 11 L/min.
> SpO2: Corrected.
> Alarms: no alarms.

> **INITIAL**: You arrive at an ICU to transfer a septic patient who is intubated. The patient is a male who weighs 190 lbs and is 6'2". He has been treated with 2 L of fluids over the las 24 hours and is on no other medications. His vital signs are HR 118, BP 88/55 with no radial pulse, $SpO_2$ 88%, and $EtCO_2$ is 52. The patient is on the ventilator: SIMV- VC, RR 16, Vt 450, I:E 1:2, $FiO_2$ 0.8, PEEP 4, Vte 448, f 19, and VE 8.5.

**Step 1: BP:**     Absent/ Weak/ Present

     Corrective Action:

**Step 2: Acidosis**: Present/ Suspected/ Possible/ Absent

     Target VE: _____
         IBW: (2.3)(___ inches > 60 inches) + 50 or 45.5 = ___
         ITV: (6-8 cc)(IBW) = _____
         RR: VE _____ / ITV _____ = RR _____

        PEEP: _____
          I:E: _____
          $FiO_2$: _____

**Step 3: Patient/ Ventilator Synchrony:**
     Below are some possible settings and findings. If the provided values do not match, provide the corrective action.

     $VE_{EXPECTED}$ _9.2_ vs. $VE_{ACTUAL}$ _9.1_    Match? Yes/ No

        Corrective Action:

     RR _16_ vs. f _16_    Match? Yes/ No

        Corrective Action:

     Vt _575_ vs. Vte _570_    Match? Yes/ No

        Corrective Action:

     PIP: _22_ Pplat: _17_    Under normal safe limits? Yes/ No

**UPDATE 1**: Your patient's vital signs and measured vent data are HR 107, BP 108/64 with a weak radial pulse, SpO2 92%, and EtCO2 is 48. The patient's ventilator settings, findings, and vital signs are: RR 16, Vt 575, I:E 1:2, VE 9.1, f 16, SpO2 92, EtCO2 48, PIP 22, Pplat 17, Vte 572, and AutoPEEP 0.

**Changes in sedation/ pain medication/ paralysis needed?** Yes/ No

If YES, explain why:

**High pressure an issue?** Yes/ No

If YES, can you r/o the DOPE acronym?

If you cannot r/o DOPE, did you switch to PC? Yes/ No

Rationale/ Notes:

**Do you need to correct minute ventilation?** Yes/ No

If so, which require changing? _____ RR/ _____TV/ _____PC

Rationale/ Notes:

**Do you need to correct the oxygenation?** Yes/ No

If so, which require correction? _____ FiO2/ _____ PEEP

Rationale/ Notes:

> **UPDATE 2**: Your patient now presents with the following vent settings, findings, and vital signs HR 102, BP 112/70 with a strong radial pulse, SpO2 97%, and EtCO2 is 41, RR 18, Vt 575, I:E 1:2, VE 10.3, PIP 21, Pplat 18, Vte 573, and AutoPEEP 0.

**Changes in sedation/ pain medication/ paralysis needed?** Yes/ No

    If YES, explain why:


**High pressure an issue?** Yes/ No

    If YES, can you r/o the DOPE acronym?

    If you cannot r/o DOPE, did you switch to PC? Yes/ No

    Rationale/ Notes:


**Do you need to correct minute ventilation?** Yes/ No

    If so, which require changing? \_\_\_\_ RR/ \_\_\_\_TV/ \_\_\_\_PC

    Rationale/ Notes:


**Do you need to correct the oxygenation?** Yes/ No

    If so, which require correction? \_\_\_\_ FiO2/ \_\_\_\_ PEEP

    Rationale/ Notes:

## Case #3: Explanation and Rationale

### General Impression:

---

**Initial Rationale:**
BP: hypotensive, so admin fluids (500cc to 1L is a good starting point).
Acidosis: Potentially present from an increased EtCO2. Additionally, hypercapnia can worsen once perfusion is restored. EtCO2 52: so increase VE to at least 9 L/min on the first change. This VE needs to be higher than normal until the CO2 is closer to normal.
Sedation: sedation is warranted in this case, so consider a sedative that doesn't cause significant drops in blood pressure, like fentanyl or ketamine.
Expected VE: 7.5 L/min; Measured VE: 7.5 L/min
Oxygenation: SpO2 88%--> increase FiO2 initially up to 1.0.
Actions needed to sync: none needed. Settings and monitored data match pretty closely.

---

**UPDATE 1 Rationale:**
EtCO2: Still a little high- but improved. Fix: increase minute ventilation (increase RR or Vt).
SpO2: improved from the increased FiO2. This improved SpO2 is still but not optimal. Fix: increase the PEEP to 5 or 6.
Alarms: none.

---

**UPDATE 2 Rationale:**
EtCO2: Corrected.
SpO2: Corrected.
Alarms: no alarms.

---

**Case# 4**                                      Date: _____

INITIAL: You and your partner have arrived at a small ER to transport a patient to a cath lab for the inferior AMI. The patient is a male who is 57 y/o, 200 lbs, and 5'11'. The patient had been talking until 10 minutes prior to your arrival. At that point, the patient passed out and was intubated. He has been treated fentanyl, rocuronium, morphine, ASA, and nitroglycerine. His vital signs are HR 92, BP 143/80 with a strong radial pulse, SpO2 87%, and EtCO2 is 55. (+) radial and carotid pulses. The patient is being ventilated via bag valve mask at a rate of 22/min.

**Step 1: BP:**    Absent/ Weak/ Present

    Corrective Action:

**Step 2: Acidosis**: Present/ Suspected/ Possible/ Absent

    Target VE: _____
        IBW: (2.3)(___ inches > 60 inches) + 50 or 45.5 = ___
        ITV: (6-8 cc)(IBW) = _____
        RR: VE _____ / ITV _____ = RR _____

        PEEP: _____
        I:E: _____
        FiO2: _____

**Step 3: Patient/ Ventilator Synchrony:**
    Below are some possible settings and findings. If the provided values do not match, provide the corrective action.

    $VE_{EXPECTED}$ _8.9_ vs. $VE_{ACTUAL}$ _6.6_    Match?  Yes/ No

        Corrective Action:

    RR _17_ vs. f _17_    Match?  Yes/ No

        Corrective Action:

    Vt _525_ vs. Vte _390_    Match?  Yes/ No

        Corrective Action:

PIP: __18__  Pplat: __13__   Under normal safe limits? Yes/ No

**Case# 4**                                                    **UPDATE 1**

---
**UPDATE 1**: Your patient's vital signs and measured vent data are HR 93, BP 138/74 with a radial pulse, SpO2 97%, EtCO2 60, RR 17, Vt 525, Vte 390, f 17, I:E 1:2, VE 6.6, PIP 18, pPlat 13, and AutoPEEP 0.

---

**Changes in sedation/ pain medication/ paralysis needed?**  Yes/ No

    If YES, explain why:

**High pressure an issue?**  Yes/ No

    If YES, can you r/o the DOPE acronym?

    If you cannot r/o DOPE, did you switch to PC?  Yes/ No

    Rationale/ Notes:

**Do you need to correct minute ventilation?**  Yes/ No

    If so, which require changing? _____ RR/ ____TV/ ____PC

    Rationale/ Notes:

**Do you need to correct the oxygenation?**  Yes/ No

    If so, which require correction? _____ FiO2/ _____ PEEP

    Rationale/ Notes:

**UPDATE 2**: Your patient now presents with the following vent settings, findings, and vital signs HR 89, BP 141/70 with a radial pulse, SpO2 98%, and EtCO2 is 49, RR 17, Vt 525, I:E 1:2, f 17, VE 10.3, PIP 18, Pplat 14, Vte 520, and AutoPEEP 0.

**Changes in sedation/ pain medication/ paralysis needed?**  Yes/ No

> If YES, explain why:


**High pressure an issue?**  Yes/ No

> If YES, can you r/o the DOPE acronym?

> If you cannot r/o DOPE, did you switch to PC?  Yes/ No

> Rationale/ Notes:


**Do you need to correct minute ventilation?**  Yes/ No

> If so, which require changing?  _____ RR/ ____TV/ ____PC

> Rationale/ Notes:


**Do you need to correct the oxygenation?**  Yes/ No

> If so, which require correction?  _____ FiO2/ _____ PEEP

> Rationale/ Notes:

## Case #4: Explanation and Rationale

**General Impression**:

---

**Initial Rationale**:
BP: adequate.
Acidosis: Potentially present from an increased EtCO2. Additionally, hypercapnia can worsen once perfusion is restored.
Target VE: most likely- begin at 9L/min or 10 L/min
IBW: 75.3, or 75 kg
ITV: 525
RR: (target VE/ ITV=RR); 9000/525= RR 17 or 10000/ 525= 19
I:E 1:2 (no evidence of bronchospasm and patient isn't a pediatric)
FiO2: 1.0 (we are initiating, so start high and titrate down as quickly as the SpO2 allows)
PEEP: 5 cmH2O (start at this upper end of normal)
Actions needed to sync: Vte is way lower than Vt setting. Rule out leak, then increase the Vt setting so that Vte rises to the desired level- titrate to effect. Watch PIP with each increase in Vt setting. Closely monitor Vte also.

---

**UPDATE 1 Rationale:**
EtCO2: this has increased since applying the mechanical ventilator. Here, the Vte is 390 when the set Vt is 525, therefore, there is either a leak or a dead space problem. Check pilot bulb and gurgling coming from oropharynx- if the pilot bulb is inflated and there isn't gurgling, then leak isn't likely. Assume a dead space problem once you rule out leak. Fix: increase the Vt setting (increase from 525 to 750). As you increase this setting, monitor the PIP to ensure dangerously high pressures are not reached. We are increasing the set Vt to overcome the dead space in the transport ventilator circuit, which helps us achieve our desired measured minute ventilation.
SpO2: corrected.
Alarms: none.

---

**UPDATE 2 Rationale**:
EtCO2: improved, but still have a little work to do. Increase the minute ventilation slightly by increasing the RR (by 1-2 breaths per minute) or the Vt (by 50 or 100 cc per breath).
SpO2: Corrected.
Alarms: no alarms.

**Case# 5**                                        Date: _____

> **INITIAL**: You arrive at an ICU where your patient has suffered a caustic ingestion of bleach. The patient is a 22 y/o who was attempting to commit suicide. The patient is in a 2 bed ICU in a small town hospital awaiting transfer to a larger regional center, is intubated, 6'4", and male. The weighs 190 lbs. His vital signs are HR 101, BP 110/72 with a radial pulse, SpO2 84%, and EtCO2 is 32. The patient is on the ventilator: SIMV- VC, RR 20, Vt 550, I:E 1:2, FiO2 0.8, PEEP 4, Vte 540, f 20, and VE 10.8.

**Step 1: BP:**    Absent/ Weak/ Present

    Corrective Action:

**Step 2: Acidosis**: Present/ Suspected/ Possible/ Absent

    Target VE: _____
        IBW: (2.3)(___ inches > 60 inches) + 50 or 45.5 = ___
        ITV: (6-8 cc)(IBW) = _____
        RR: VE _____ / ITV _____ = RR _____

        PEEP: _____
          I:E: _____
        FiO2: _____

**Step 3: Patient/ Ventilator Synchrony:**
    Below are some possible settings and findings. If the provided values do not match, provide the corrective action.

    VE$_{EXPECTED}$ _9.9_ vs. VE$_{ACTUAL}$ _9.7_    Match?  Yes/ No

        Corrective Action:

    RR _18_ vs. f _18_    Match?  Yes/ No

        Corrective Action:

    Vt _550_ vs. Vte _540_    Match?  Yes/ No

        Corrective Action:

    PIP: _17_ Pplat: _13_   Under normal safe limits? Yes/ No

**Changes in sedation/ pain medication/ paralysis needed?** Yes/ No

If YES, explain why:

**High pressure an issue?** Yes/ No

If YES, can you r/o the DOPE acronym?

If you cannot r/o DOPE, did you switch to PC? Yes/ No

Rationale/ Notes:

**Do you need to correct minute ventilation?** Yes/ No

If so, which require changing? _____ RR/ _____TV/ _____PC

Rationale/ Notes:

**Do you need to correct the oxygenation?** Yes/ No

If so, which require correction? _____ FiO2/ _____ PEEP

Rationale/ Notes:

> **UPDATE 2**: En route to your destination, you receive a high pressure alarm. Your patient now presents with the following vent settings, findings, and vital signs HR 108, BP 115/73 with a strong radial pulse, SpO2 84%, and EtCO2 is 56, RR 18, Vt 550, I:E 1:2, VE 9.7, Vte 540, and PIP 55, pPlat 51, AutoPEEP 0. No tube dislodgement or obstruction noted.

**Changes in sedation/ pain medication/ paralysis needed?** Yes/ No

    If YES, explain why:


**High pressure an issue?** Yes/ No

    If YES, can you r/o the DOPE acronym?

    If you cannot r/o DOPE, did you switch to PC? Yes/ No

    Rationale/ Notes:


**Do you need to correct minute ventilation?** Yes/ No

    If so, which require changing? _____ RR/ _____TV/ _____PC

    Rationale/ Notes:


**Do you need to correct the oxygenation?** Yes/ No

    If so, which require correction? _____ FiO2/ _____ PEEP

    Rationale/ Notes:

## Case #5: Explanation and Rationale

**General Impression**:

---

**Initial Rationale**:
BP: adequate.
Acidosis/ Ventilation: in this case, the medical team is moving too much $CO_2$ resulting in an $EtCO_2$ of 32, therefore, minute ventilation needs to be reduced. It only needs to be reduced a little bit, so a change in RR of 2 breaths/min or a change of Vt by 500cc- 1000cc would be a great starting point.
Oxygenation: $SpO_2$ 88%--> increase $FiO_2$ initially to 1.0.
Sedation: sedation is looks to be sufficient at this time since the set RR matches the monitored f.
Expected VE: 11 L/min; Measured VE: 10.8 L/min. These are close enough to be considered equivalent.
Actions needed to sync: none needed. Settings and monitored data match pretty closely.

---

**UPDATE 1 Rationale:**
$EtCO_2$: corrected.
$SpO_2$: corrected.
Alarms: none.

---

**UPDATE 2 Rationale**:
$EtCO_2$: now, we have a higher $EtCO_2$ so we need to increase minute ventilation. To achieve this, increase RR or Vt. Small incremental changes provide valuable feedback to the clinician.
$SpO_2$: Now, $SpO_2$ is low, so and increase in PEEP IS warranted. Increase by 2 or 3 $cmH_2O$ at a time.
Alarms: We have a high pressure alarm, therefore, we need to investigate the DOPE acronym and then investigate PIP vs PPlat pressures if DOPE is ruled out.

**Case# 6**                                        Date: _____

---

**INITIAL**: En route to your destination, you receive a high pressure alarm.
You have ruled out the DOPE acronym and have discovered that the
patient's PIP is 56 and the Pplat is 52. Your patient is a 250 lbs male and has
the following vent settings, findings, and vital signs HR 112, BP 105/65 with
a weak radial pulse, SpO2 86%, and EtCO2 is 48, RR 18, Vt 625, I:E 1:2,
PEEP 6, VE 11.1, PIP 57, Pplat 53, Vte 621, f 18, and AutoPEEP 0.

---

**Step 1: BP:**    Absent/ Weak/ Present

   Corrective Action:

**Step 2: Acidosis**: Present/ Suspected/ Possible/ Absent

   Target VE: _____
        IBW: (2.3)(___ inches > 60 inches) + 50 or 45.5 = ___
        ITV: (6-8 cc)(IBW) = _____
        RR: VE _____ / ITV _____ = RR _____

        PEEP: _____
         I:E: _____
         FiO2: _____

## Step 3: Patient/ Ventilator Synchrony:
Below are some possible settings and findings. If the provided values do not
match, provide the corrective action.

   VE$_{EXPECTED}$ _n/a_ vs. VE$_{ACTUAL}$ _n/a_   Match?  Yes/ No

      Corrective Action:

   RR _18_ vs. f _18_   Match?  Yes/ No

      Corrective Action:

   Vt _n/a- on PC_ vs. Vte _615_   ~~Match?  Yes/ No~~

      Corrective Action:

   PIP: _27_  Pplat: _n/a- on PC_   Under normal safe limits? Yes/ No

120

**UPDATE 1**: Your patient's vital signs and measured vent data are HR 100, BP 109/72 with a radial pulse, SpO2 89%, and EtCO2 is 37. The patient's ventilator settings, findings, and vital signs are: SIMV- PC 19, RR 18, I:E 1:2, FiO2 1.0, PEEP 8, Vte 615, f 18, VE 11.0, PIP 27, and AutoPEEP 0.

**Changes in sedation/ pain medication/ paralysis needed?**  Yes/ No

   If YES, explain why:

**High pressure an issue?**  Yes/ No

   If YES, can you r/o the DOPE acronym?

   If you cannot r/o DOPE, did you switch to PC?  Yes/ No

   Rationale/ Notes:

**Do you need to correct minute ventilation?**  Yes/ No

   If so, which require changing?  _____ RR/ _____TV/ _____PC

   Rationale/ Notes:

**Do you need to correct the oxygenation?**  Yes/ No

   If so, which require correction?  _____ FiO2/ _____ PEEP

   Rationale/ Notes:

**UPDATE 2**: Your patient now presents with the following vent settings, findings, and vital signs: SIMV- PC 20, RR 41, I:E 1:2, FiO2 1.0, PEEP 20, Vte 275, PIP 40, and AutoPEEP 3. HR 101, BP 105/69 with a radial pulse, SpO2 93%, and EtCO2 is 39.

**Changes in sedation/ pain medication/ paralysis needed?**  Yes/ No

If YES, explain why:

**High pressure an issue?**  Yes/ No

If YES, can you r/o the DOPE acronym?

If you cannot r/o DOPE, did you switch to PC?  Yes/ No

Rationale/ Notes:

**Do you need to correct minute ventilation?**  Yes/ No

If so, which require changing?  _____ RR/ _____TV/ _____PC

Rationale/ Notes:

**Do you need to correct the oxygenation?**  Yes/ No

If so, which require correction?  _____ FiO2/ _____ PEEP

Rationale/ Notes:

# Case #6: Explanation and Rationale

## General Impression:

**Initial Rationale:**
BP: adequate.
Acidosis/ Ventilation: there has been a significant change in the patient status. The patient is literally developing ARDS or acute lung injury (ALI) in front of your eyes. The high pressures, specifically the high Pplat pressures, indicate slung damage. Immediately we should switch from volume control ventilation to pressure control. To do this, we need to set the pressure control setting to 20 cmH2O and adopt the PEEP of 6. Adding 20 plus 6 we get 26, therefore, our expected PIP is 26 after switching to pressure control ventilation. This ensures we will no longer damage lung tissue with mechanical ventilations. Next, it is important to titrate the pressure control setting to achieve a Vte similar and a little higher than what the patient was ventilating when their EtCO2 was in normal range. We will still need to make on the fly changes based on the EtCO2 as the flight/ call progresses.
Oxygenation: SpO2 86%--> increase PEEP to 8 or 9 cmH2O.
Sedation: sedation is looks to be sufficient at this time since the set RR matches the monitored f.
Expected VE: 11.2 L/min; Measured VE: 11.1 L/min. These are close enough to be considered equivalent.
Actions needed to sync: none needed. Settings and monitored data match pretty closely.

**UPDATE 1 Rationale:**
EtCO2: corrected.
SpO2: Still low, but improving. At this point you should realize that PEEP is directly supporting your oxygenation and you will most likely need more with an ARDS patient. Your plan of care should include 1) increasing your PEEP to 10, 2) obtain medical control orders for up to 20 or PEEP, and 3) obtain medical control orders to reverse the I:E ratio should you get to 20 of PEEP and still need more 'firepower.' Assume you have all these orders approved for the next update. Fix: max PEEP at 20 cmH2O.
Alarms: none.

**UPDATE 2 Rationale:**
EtCO2: Corrected. You'll notice the frequency (f) is very high and the Vte is low. Remember, those two parameters multiplied together determine the minute ventilation. Also recall that RR isn't dangerous until we start to breaths stack, but if we are trying to cause AutoPEEP (like in patients who benefit from reverse I:E ratio) then there is no danger. The RR setting is so high because when you increase PEEP to beyond 10 cmH2O you begin to reduce available space (or tidal volume) in the lung, and this can be observed as a drop in Vte when PEEP is increased. To maintain a minute volume consistent with the needs of the patient (EtCO2 between 35-45 mmHg) higher rates will be needed to overcome the smaller Vte (caused by higher PEEPs).
SpO2: the max PEEP is improving the patient significantly but there needs to be a little more support added. Reverse the I:E ratio here (2:1 setting on the ventilator). This is create a bi-level PAP by establishing constant and maximal CPAP (PEEP) with an inspiratory PAP as well (executed by the PC setting).
Alarms: none.

---

**INITIAL**: You are transporting a hypotensive multi-system trauma patient. The patient is a 6'5" male. He has been treated with 2 L of fluids and 3 units of packed red blood cells. His vital signs are HR 107, BP 87/55 without a radial pulse, SpO2 89%, and EtCO2 is 26. The patient is on the ventilator: SIMV- VC, RR 12, Vt 500, I:E 1:2, FiO2 0.6, PEEP 3, Vte 490, f 12, and VE 5.8.

---

**Step 1: BP:**    Absent/ Weak/ Present

Corrective Action:

**Step 2: Acidosis**: Present/ Suspected/ Possible/ Absent

Target VE: _____
    IBW: (2.3)(___ inches > 60 inches) + 50 or 45.5 = ___
    ITV: (6-8 cc)(IBW) = _____
    RR: VE _____ / ITV _____ = RR _____

PEEP: _____
    I:E: _____
    FiO2: _____

## Step 3: Patient/ Ventilator Synchrony:
Below are some possible settings and findings. If the provided values do not match, provide the corrective action.

$VE_{EXPECTED}$ __5.8__ vs. $VE_{ACTUAL}$ __5.8__    Match?  Yes/ No

    Corrective Action:

RR __12__ vs. f __12__    Match?  Yes/ No

    Corrective Action:

Vt __490__ vs. Vte __500__    Match?  Yes/ No

    Corrective Action:

PIP: __19__ Pplat: __17__    Under normal safe limits? Yes/ No

**UPDATE 1**: Your patient's vital signs and measured vent data are now HR 103, BP 92/66 without a radial pulse, SpO2 91%, and EtCO2 is 28. The patient's ventilator settings, findings, and vital signs are: RR 16, Vt 500, f 16, I:E 1:2, VE 7.8, PIP 19, SpO2 92, EtCO2 48, Pplat 17, Vte 490, and AutoPEEP 0. You administer another 750 cc LR bolus.

**Changes in sedation/ pain medication/ paralysis needed?**  Yes/ No

If YES, explain why:

**High pressure an issue?**  Yes/ No

If YES, can you r/o the DOPE acronym?

If you cannot r/o DOPE, did you switch to PC?  Yes/ No

Rationale/ Notes:

**Do you need to correct minute ventilation?**  Yes/ No

If so, which require changing?  _____ RR/ _____TV/ _____PC

Rationale/ Notes:

**Do you need to correct the oxygenation?**  Yes/ No

If so, which require correction?  _____ FiO2/ _____ PEEP

Rationale/ Notes:

---

**UPDATE 2**: The patient has now been treated. There are no alarms currently sounding. Current vent settings are volume control in A/C mode with RR 18, I:E 1:2, Vt 500, PEEP 5, and FiO2 of 1.0. Your patient's vital signs and measured vent data are BP 112/70 with strong radial pulses, HR 103, RR vent assisted at 18, SpO2 98%, EtCO2 is 41, VE 8.8, f 18, Vte 490, PIP 20, Pplat 16, and AutoPEEP 0.

---

**Changes in sedation/ pain medication/ paralysis needed?**  Yes/ No

    If YES, explain why:


**High pressure an issue?**  Yes/ No

    If YES, can you r/o the DOPE acronym?

    If you cannot r/o DOPE, did you switch to PC?  Yes/ No

    Rationale/ Notes:


**Do you need to correct minute ventilation?**  Yes/ No

    If so, which require changing?  _____ RR/ ____TV/ ____PC

    Rationale/ Notes:


**Do you need to correct the oxygenation?**  Yes/ No

    If so, which require correction?  _____ FiO2/ _____ PEEP

    Rationale/ Notes:

## Case #7: Explanation and Rationale

**General Impression**:

---

**Initial Rationale**:
BP: Compromised- hypotensive.
Acidosis: Unknown here, however, luckily he is already on the ventilator and we can just "surf." If the patient is acidotic, with the low EtCO2 as well, we may need to avoid in increasing EtCO2. It's important to get BP up so we have accurate vital sign data.
Target VE: hold as is until BP is corrected or we receive an ABG. Currently the VE is 5.8.
IBW: 89.1, or 90 kg
ITV: 630 (90 kg x 7 cc/kg of tidal volume)
RR: Already on vent: 12/min with f of 12/min as well- he is well sedated.
I:E 1:2 (no evidence of bronchospasm and patient isn't a pediatric)
FiO2: 0.6- need to increase.
PEEP: 3- need to increase.
Actions needed to sync: none needed. Settings and monitored data match pretty closely.

---

**UPDATE 1 Rationale:**
EtCO2: Remains low. BP has improved, but no strong radial pule yet- more fluids needed.
SpO2: Still low, but improved. Continue to increase FiO2 or PEEP.
Alarms: No alarms.

---

**UPDATE 2 Rationale**:
EtCO2: Corrected.
SpO2: Corrected.
Alarms: no alarms.

**Case# 8**                                          Date: _____

> **INITIAL**: You arrive at a small hospital to pick up a patient who is suffering anaphylaxis. The patient was stung by a bee earlier this afternoon and had been intubated to protect his airway. The patient is a 6'0" male. He has been treated with 2 L of fluids and is on neosynepherine. His vital signs are HR 99, BP 110/60 with radial pulse, SpO2 97%, and EtCO2 is 33. The patient is on the ventilator: SIMV- VC, RR 14, Vt 540, I:E 1:2, FiO2 0.8, PEEP 4, Vte 535, f 22, and VE 11.7.

**Step 1: BP:**    Absent/ Weak/ Present

    Corrective Action:

**Step 2: Acidosis**: Present/ Suspected/ Possible/ Absent

    Target VE: _____
        IBW: (2.3)(___ inches > 60 inches) + 50 or 45.5 = ___
        ITV: (6-8 cc)(IBW) = _____
        RR: VE _____ / ITV _____ = RR _____

        PEEP: _____
        I:E: _____
        FiO2: _____

**Step 3: Patient/ Ventilator Synchrony:**
    Below are some possible settings and findings. If the provided values do not match, provide the corrective action.

    $VE_{EXPECTED}$ _7.5_ vs. $VE_{ACTUAL}$ _11.7_    Match?  Yes/ No

    Corrective Action:

    RR _17_ vs. f _26_    Match?  Yes/ No

    Corrective Action:

    Vt _540_ vs. Vte _535_    Match?  Yes/ No

    Corrective Action:

    PIP: _17_ Pplat: _13_    Under normal safe limits? Yes/ No

**UPDATE 1**: Your patient's vital signs and measured vent data are HR 97, BP 108/64 with a weak radial pulse, SpO2 99%, and EtCO2 is 46. The patient's ventilator settings, findings, and vital signs are: SIMV- VC, RR 14, Vt 540, I:E 1:2, FiO2 0.8, PEEP 4, Vte 535, f 19, and VE 10.1, PIP 22, Pplat 17, and AutoPEEP 0.

**Changes in sedation/ pain medication/ paralysis needed?** Yes/ No

    If YES, explain why:

**High pressure an issue?** Yes/ No

    If YES, can you r/o the DOPE acronym?

    If you cannot r/o DOPE, did you switch to PC? Yes/ No

    Rationale/ Notes:

**Do you need to correct minute ventilation?** Yes/ No

    If so, which require changing? _____ RR/ _____TV/ _____PC

    Rationale/ Notes:

**Do you need to correct the oxygenation?** Yes/ No

    If so, which require correction? _____ FiO2/ _____ PEEP

    Rationale/ Notes:

**UPDATE 2**: Minute ventilation has been corrected by sedating the patient and returning the frequency back to match the set RR. There is no alarms currently sounding. Current vent settings are volume control in SIMV mode with RR 16, I:E 1:2, Vt 540, PEEP 5, and FiO2 of 1.0. Your patient's vital signs and measured vent data are BP 118/84 with strong radial pulses, HR 99, SpO2 98%, EtCO2 is 44, VE 8.5, f 16, Vte 535, PIP 19, Pplat 14, and AutoPEEP 0.

**Changes in sedation/ pain medication/ paralysis needed?** Yes/ No

    If YES, explain why:

**High pressure an issue?** Yes/ No

    If YES, can you r/o the DOPE acronym?

    If you cannot r/o DOPE, did you switch to PC? Yes/ No

    Rationale/ Notes:

**Do you need to correct minute ventilation?** Yes/ No

    If so, which require changing? _____ RR/ _____TV/ _____PC

    Rationale/ Notes:

**Do you need to correct the oxygenation?** Yes/ No

    If so, which require correction? _____ FiO2/ _____ PEEP

    Rationale/ Notes:

## Case #8: Explanation and Rationale

### General Impression:

> **Initial Rationale:**
> <u>BP</u>: Adequate (appears adequate)
> <u>Acidosis</u>: None suspected at this time.
> <u>Target VE</u>: Already in a vent- "vent surf"
> <u>IBW</u>: 77.6, or round to78 kg
> <u>ITV</u>: 546 (78 kg x 7 cc/kg of tidal volume)
> <u>RR</u>: (target VE/ ITV=RR); 9000/546= RR 16 or 10000/ 560= 16.4, or 16. But remember, he is already on a vent- "vent surf".
> <u>I:E</u> 1:2 could be fine, but you could consider that bronchoconstriction could be happening and monitor the EtCO2 waveform and AutoPEEP for evidence of bronchospasm.
> <u>FiO2</u>: 0.8- Adequate since SpO2 is > 94%
> <u>PEEP</u>: 4 cmH2O- Adequate since SpO2 is > 94%
> <u>Corrective Actions</u>: The f and VE are both high. Sedate the patient or increase vent sensitivity to return VE and f back to the desired ranges.

> **UPDATE 1 Rationale:**
> <u>EtCO2</u>: Improved, but now pushed past the normal upper limit. Slightly increase minute ventilation..
> <u>SpO2</u>: Normal.
> <u>Alarms</u>: high minute ventilation. Cause: increased frequency (f) of 19/min compared to the preset RR of 14. The f of 19 x Vte of 535 equals our measured VE of 10.1 L/min, and therefore strongly suggests the rationale of high minute ventilation due to high frequency most likely from the patient being under sedated. Also, a low sensitivity causes the vent to be triggered if vibrations are too high. Fix: 1) increase sensitivity setting and 2) sedate and/or paralyze the patient to prevent patient initiated attempts.

> **UPDATE 2 Rationale:**
> <u>EtCO2</u>: Corrected.
> <u>SpO2</u>: Corrected.
> <u>Alarms</u>: no alarms.

**Case# 9**　　　　　　　　　　　　　　　　　　Date: _____

| INITIAL: Your pediatric patient is 3 months old and 6 kg with pneumonia. His vital signs are HR 144, BP pink extremities with normal capillary refill to the nailbeds, RR assisted at 30/min via BVM, SpO2 84%, and EtCO2 is 58. |
| --- |

**Step 1: BP:**　　Absent/ Weak/ Present

　　Corrective Action:

**Step 2: Acidosis**: Present/ Suspected/ Possible/ Absent

　　Target VE: _____
　　　　IBW: (9 + months in age) / 2= ___
　　　　ITV: (6-8 cc)(IBW) = _____
　　　　RR: VE _____ / ITV _____ = RR _____

　　　　PEEP: _____
　　　　I:E: _____
　　　　FiO2: _____

## Step 3: Patient/ Ventilator Synchrony:
Below are some possible settings and findings. If the provided values do not match, provide the corrective action.

　　$VE_{EXPECTED}$ _n/a_ vs. $VE_{ACTUAL}$ _n/a_　Match?　Yes/ No

　　　　Corrective Action:

　　RR _35_ vs. f _38_　　Match?　Yes/ No

　　　　Corrective Action:

　　Vt _n/a- on PC_ vs. Vte _90_　~~Match? Yes/ No~~

　　　　Corrective Action:

　　PIP: _24_　Pplat: _n/a- on PC_　Under normal safe limits? Yes/ No

> **UPDATE 1**: Your patient's vital signs and measured vent data are BP pink extremities with normal capillary refill to the nailbeds, HR 138, RR vent assisted at 35, SpO2 90%, EtCO2 is 51, PC 18, VE 3.4, f 38, PEEP 5, Vte 90, PIP 24, and AutoPEEP 0.

**Changes in sedation/ pain medication/ paralysis needed?** Yes/ No

    If YES, explain why:

**High pressure an issue?** Yes/ No

    If YES, can you r/o the DOPE acronym?

    If you cannot r/o DOPE, did you switch to PC? Yes/ No

    Rationale/ Notes:

**Do you need to correct minute ventilation?** Yes/ No

    If so, which require changing? _____ RR/ _____TV/ _____PC

    Rationale/ Notes:

**Do you need to correct the oxygenation?** Yes/ No

    If so, which require correction? _____ FiO2/ _____ PEEP

    Rationale/ Notes:

**UPDATE 2**: Your patient's vital signs and measured vent data are now BP
pink extremities with normal capillary refill to the nailbeds, HR 138, RR vent
assisted at 35, SpO2 96%, EtCO2 is 47, PC 20, VE 4.0, f 35, PEEP 7, Vte
115, PIP 24, and AutoPEEP 0.

**Changes in sedation/ pain medication/ paralysis needed?**  Yes/ No

   If YES, explain why:


**High pressure an issue?**  Yes/ No

   If YES, can you r/o the DOPE acronym?

   If you cannot r/o DOPE, did you switch to PC?  Yes/ No

   Rationale/ Notes:


**Do you need to correct minute ventilation?**  Yes/ No

   If so, which require changing?  _____ RR/ _____TV/ _____PC

   Rationale/ Notes:


**Do you need to correct the oxygenation?**  Yes/ No

   If so, which require correction?  _____ FiO2/ _____ PEEP

   Rationale/ Notes:

## Case #9: Explanation and Rationale

**General Impression**:

---

**Initial Rationale**:
BP: Appears pink (adequate)
Acidosis: potentially present (high EtCO2)
Target VE: most likely- begin at 2L/min or 3 L/min
IBW: 6 kg
ITV: 42 (6 kg x 7 cc/kg of tidal volume)
RR: (target VE/ ITV=RR); 2000/42= RR 47. Since this seems higher, monitor AutoPEEP often and lengthen the I:E ratio if the AutoPEEP is ever 1 or 2 cmH2O.
PC: 20 cmH2O
I:E 1:5 (pediatric patient)
FiO2: 1.0 (we are initiating, so start high and titrate down as quickly as the SpO2 allows)
PEEP: 5 cmH2O ( start at this upper end of normal)
Corrective Actions: Their f is a little high. Perhaps consider sedating or ruling out a sensitivity problem.

---

**UPDATE 1 Rationale:**
EtCO2: Reduced, but still elevated. Minute ventilation will need to be increased to blow off more EtCO2.
SpO2: Still low, but improved. Continue to increase FiO2 or PEEP.
Alarms: None.
The patient has a f that is 3 breaths higher than the set RR. This indicates the patient could be waking up, therefore, sedation is warranted in this case.

---

**UPDATE 2 Rationale**:
EtCO2: The EtCO2 is still a little high, but improving. Increase minute ventilation just a little bit more (increase RR or PC in this case).
SpO2: Corrected.
Alarms: no alarms.

> **INITIAL**: You have a patient who is awake and having shortness of breath. The patient has CHF and is a 6'2" male. His vital signs are HR 94, BP 143/92, RR 26, SpO2 91%, and EtCO2 is 42.

## Step 1: BP:    Absent/ Weak/ Present

Corrective Action:

## Step 2: Acidosis: Present/ Suspected/ Possible/ Absent

## BPAP SETTINGS:

IPAP (PS): _____

EPAP (PEEP): _____

## Step 3: Patient/ Ventilator Synchrony:

Below are some possible settings and findings. If the provided values do not match, provide the corrective action.

$VE_{EXPECTED}$ _n/a_ vs. $VE_{ACTUAL}$ _n/a_    Match?  Yes/ No

Corrective Action:

RR _n/a_ vs. f _n/a_    Match?  Yes/ No

Corrective Action:

Vt _n/a_ vs. Vte _n/a_    Match?  Yes/ No

Corrective Action:

PIP: _n/a_ Pplat: _n/a_  Under normal safe limits? Yes/ No

> **UPDATE 1**: Your patient's vital signs and measured vent data are HR 101, BP 144/90 with a strong radial pulse, SpO2 92%, and EtCO2 is 50. The patient is still calm but is becoming increasingly short of breath.

**Changes in sedation/ pain medication/ paralysis needed?** Yes/ No

    If YES, explain why:

**High pressure an issue?** Yes/ No

    If YES, can you r/o the DOPE acronym?

    If you cannot r/o DOPE, did you switch to PC? Yes/ No

    Rationale/ Notes:

**Do you need to correct minute ventilation?** Yes/ No

    If so, which require changing? _____ RR/ _____TV/ _____PC

    Rationale/ Notes:

**Do you need to correct the oxygenation?** Yes/ No

    If so, which require correction? _____ FiO2/ _____ PEEP

    Rationale/ Notes:

**UPDATE 2**: Your patient now presents with the following findings and vital signs HR 110, BP 143/89 with a strong radial pulse, SpO2 88%, and EtCO2 is 56, and RR 24.

**Step 1: BP:**    Absent/ Weak/ Present

Corrective Action:

**Step 2: Acidosis**: Present/ Suspected/ Possible/ Absent

Target VE: _____
    IBW: (2.3)(___ inches > 60 inches) + 50 or 45.5 = ___
    ITV: (6-8 cc)(IBW) = _____
    RR: VE _____ / ITV _____ = RR _____

PEEP: _____
    I:E: _____
    FiO2: _____

**Step 3: Patient/ Ventilator Synchrony**:
Below are some possible settings and findings. If the provided values do not match, provide the corrective action.

$VE_{EXPECTED}$ __9.0__ vs. $VE_{ACTUAL}$ __11.2__    Match?  Yes/ No

Corrective Action:

RR __16__ vs. f __20__    Match?  Yes/ No

Corrective Action:

Vt __575__ vs. Vte __560__    Match?  Yes/ No

Corrective Action:

PIP: __25__  Pplat: __21__   Under normal safe limits? Yes/ No

## Case #10: Explanation and Rationale

**General Impression**:

**Initial Rationale**:
This patient should be placed on noninvasive positive pressure ventilation specifically in the CPAP mode. CPAP is preferred in this case because all we need is to fix the oxygenation problem. There is no ventilation problem at this time as reported by the end tidal $CO_2$. Had the $EtCO_2$ been high, then bi-level PAP would have been ideal since there would be both an oxygenation problem and a ventilation problem.
BP: adequate.
Acidosis/ Ventilation: no acidosis suspected at this time.
Sedation: none needed currently.
Ventilation: $EtCO_2$ normal.
Oxygenation: $SpO_2$ 91%- low. Apply CPAP by setting an EPAP to 5-6 cmH2O.

**UPDATE 1 Rationale:**
$EtCO_2$: now the end tidal is higher than before, indicating a potential impending respiratory failure. If we cannot turn them around very soon, then they'll need to be intubated. Increase the difference between the IPAP and EPAP. This can be done by making the IPAP higher, thus increasing the pressure support ability of IPAP and minute ventilation.
$SpO_2$: The $SpO_2$ has increased but by just barely. Increase the EPAP. However, be mindful that by increasing EPAP you'll decrease the difference between IPAP and EPAP. In this case to improve both oxygenation and ventilation, you'll need to increase EPAP room prove the oxygenation side and then increase the IPAP by the same value you increased EPAP plus a little extra (say 2-5 CmH2O). Also recall that the higher you set these pressures, your PIP will also go up so keep track and don't go over a PIP of 35 cmH2O to prevent barotrauma.
Alarms: none.

**UPDATE 2 Rationale**:
$EtCO_2$: increased.
$SpO_2$: decreased.
Alarms: no alarms.
It's time to intubate this patient. The patient's BP is sufficient and the patient is potentially acidotic (from the high $EtCO_2$). The patient is 6'2" therefore he has an IBW of 82 kg (14 x 2.3 then added to 50). Tidal volume factor of 7 cc/kg multiplied to his IBW results in 575 cc. If we target a minute ventilation of 9 L/min (because he is acidotic) then we divide 575 cc into this 9 L/min resulting in an RR of 16. We can start the $FiO_2$ at 1.0, PEEP of 5, and I:E ratio of 1:2. From this point you would want to surf $SpO_2$ and $EtCO_2$ to try to titrate these vital signs into normal ranges.

## PRACTICE SESSION #1:

1.  Their expected minute ventilation is 7 L/min. This is obtained from the observed RR of 14 breaths/min multiplied by the estimated tidal volume (14 x 500 = 7000, or 7 liters).
2.  Their expected minute ventilation is 8.1 L/min. This is obtained from the observed RR of 18 breaths/min multiplied by the tidal volume (18 x 450 = 8100 cc, or 8.1 liters).
3.  Your patient has an $EtCO_2$ of 60, RR of 20 and a Vt of 450. Which of the following would correct the $EtCO_2$?
    a.  Lower minute ventilation
    b.  **Increase the RR to 24**
    c.  Reduce the Vt to 400
    d.  Increase the EtCO

    **Note**: The only way to change $EtCO_2$ is to increase or decrease the minute ventilation. To effect change in the $EtCO_2$ you need to change RR, Vt, or PC, and in this case we need to increase minute ventilation to reduce the $EtCO_2$, therefore, increasing the RR to 24 is the only option achieving this change.

## PRACTICE SESSION #2:

1. You are transporting an 11 month old patient with pneumonia. You intubate the patient and will now apply the mechanical ventilator. Which of the following are appropriate initial settings? Circle one: Volume or **Pressure**.

2. Your patient is a middle aged adult who presents with an AMI and is being transferred to a cath lab. The sending facility intubated your patient just prior to your arrival and is currently bagging with a BVM. Which of the following are appropriate initial settings? Circle one: **Volume** or Pressure.

3. To achieve this tidal volume you would need to increase either the PC setting or the RR. We are not given RR in this case, so I'd increase that PC by 2 cmH2O to 19 cmH2O. This would raise the Vte closer to our target Vt of 450 cc.

## PRACTICE SESSION #3:

1. Your female patient is 5'9". What is her IBW? **66.2 kg of IBW.**

2. Your male patient is 6'3" and weighs 350 pounds. What is his IBW? **84.5 kg of IBW.**

3. What is the ideal tidal volume for a 6'1" female who weighs 132 lbs? **Her IBW would be 75.4, so if you multiply this IBW by the factor for tidal volume (5-8 cc/kg) we arrive at a range of ideal tidal volume (ITV) of 377- 603 cc. Anywhere within this range would be considered ITV.**

1. What I:E ratio would you apply to a patient with a "shark fin" morphology on their EtCO2 waveform? **You would want to apply an I:E ratio with a longer E-time, such as 1:5 or 1:6 to allow for longer exhalation time. With asthma or other forms of air trapping, we see a 'shark fin' morphology on the EtCO2 graphic waveform. This indicates air trapping, therefore, we need to allow for longer E-times to allow that trapped gas to escape.**

2. Your Patient is on pressure control ventilation and the set PC is 19. Their Vte is 450 cc and their EtCO2 is 49 mmHg. What change can you make to drive this EtCO2 closer to the normal range? **To get this EtCO2 into a lower and more normal range, we need to increase the minute ventilation. To do this, recall we need to change RR, Vt, or PC. In this case we are given a PC setting, so if we increase the PC setting, say to 21 cmH2O, then the Vte should rise thus decreasing the EtCO2. Additionally, we could increase the RR, but I challenge you to start truly using the PC setting and thinking of it as a way to increase or decrease the tidal volume the patient receives.**

3. What 2 settings can be changed to correct EtCO2? **RR and Vt. Vt can be changed directly by changing the tidal volume setting (if in volume control ventilation) or indirectly by changing the PC setting (if in pressure control ventilation).**

4. What 2 settings can be changed to correct oxygenation problems? **PEEP and FiO2.**

PRACTICE SESSION #5:

1. Explain the importance of peak inspiratory pressure. **Peak inspiratory pressure (PIP) is a great indicator that something is wrong within the airway. Normally, PIP is under 35 cmH2O, so when the PIP begins to elevate it**

alerts us to look for issues within the airway that would cause an increased pressure. These would include endotracheal tube dislodgemeant, obstructions (kinked endotracheal tube, secretions in the airway, bronchospasm), tension pneumothorax, and faulty equipment. Using the DOPE acronym can remind you of these possibilities. These findings represent quick fixes to a high pressure alarm. If a high pressure alarm (high PIP) occurs and these quick fixes are not the culprit, then immediately obtain a plateau pressure.

2. Explain the importance of plateau pressure. **While the PIP is a whistle blower, it isn't specific to a particular cause of high pressure in the airway. Plateau pressure on the other hand is specific to damaging lung tissue. If the plateau pressure is ever over 30 ccH2O, then lung damage is occurring. Immediately at this point withdraw volume control ventilation and start the patient on reassure control ventilation to prevent these high pressures caused by volume control ventilation and the pulmonary pathophysiology that is preventing normal compliance of the patient's lungs.**

3. Why is mean airway pressure important in the inspiratory phase of ventilation? **The mean airway pressure is the average pressure in the lung throughout ventilation. It obviously holds open alveoli and thus increase the alveolar size as well as thins the walls of the alveoli- both add to oxygenation.**

## PRACTICE SESSION #6:

1. Explain what happens when sensitivity is set too low on the mechanical ventilator. **Sensitivity is a setting that determines how hard the patient has to breathe in to trigger a machine breath. It is measured in negative cmH2O. A sensitivity setting of 1 means the patient has to draw in a breath at only -1 cmH2O to initiate a machine breath. A sensitivity of 4 means the patient**

would have to draw down -4 cmH2O to initiate a machine breath. The A/C, SIMV, and PRVC modes provide machine breaths when the patient breeches the sensitivity threshold. So, if the sensitivity is set too low it is easy for the patient to take a breath. Additionally, vibrations in your transport vehicle could also trigger inwanted machine breaths if the sensitivity is set too low. Remember, we want to control our patients so we can in effect control their physiology. Allowing them to breathe much more that your settings would be deliberately preventing this.

2.   Describe how a mechanically ventilated breath progresses from inspiration to exhalation. **An inspiration is begun by either the patient (patient- driven breath) or because the RR dictates it's time for another breath (machine breath). Air is then advanced into the the lungs until either a pre- selected volume (volume control) or a predetermined pressure is reached (pressure control). Once either set volume or pressure is reached, then inspiration stops and exhalation is allowed. Inspiratory time also plays a role by limiting the time inspiration can occur. Exhalation is then allowed to occur. Once enough time goes by or when ever the patient attempts to take a breath, inspiration is initiated and the entire process occurs again.**

3.   How is the inspiratory phase of a mechanically initiated breath halted? **The inspiratory phase of a mechanically ventilated breath is halted once either the pre-set volume (volume controlled ventilation) or pre-set pressure (pressure control ventilation) is reached within the lungs. Once these predetermined parameters are reached, then inspiration stops and exhalation begins.**

## PRACTICE SESSION #7:

1.   How can flow rates be adjusted in the transport ventilators? **You can increase flow rates by**

accessing your ventilator's RISE TIME function. Look in the manual of your specific ventilator to learn the procedure. Rise time acts as a way for air to be advanced into the lungs either faster or slower, which is basically the function of flow rate.

2. What type of patients could benefit from lower rise times in the transport ventilators? **Patients with airway resistance problems can benefit from lower profile rise time.**

3. Your patient is breathing 12 times per minute. If you set your I-time at 1.0 second, what is your I:E ratio? **This means one second of the breath cycle is all inspiration. At a rate of 12 per minute each breath cycle would last 5 seconds, so TCT is 5 seconds (50 seconds/12 = 5 seconds). So, if the I-time is 1.0 second, then the E-time is 4.0 seconds. Therefore, the I:E ratio is simply 1:4. Now, let's say the I-time wasn't 1.0 and instead it was 1.2 seconds. Let's also assume the respiratory rate was still 12/min and therefore the TCT would also still be 5 seconds. To calculate the ratio,**

>   1. **Subtract I-time from TCT (5 − 1.2 = 3.8).**
>   2. **This gives a raw ratio of 1.2 to 3.8.**
>   3. **Divide the I-time into itself and then into the E-time:**
>       a. **1.2 / 1.2 = 1**
>       b. **3.8 / 1.2 = 3.1**
>   4. **I:E ratio is 1:3.1.**

## PRACTICE SESSION #8:

1. How can the inspiratory hold maneuver be used as a diagnostic? **The inspiratory hold maneuver provides us with the plateau pressure and therefore tells us that our selected tidal volume is either self for the patient (if pPlat is < 30 cmH2O) or if it is dangerous (indicated by a pPlat over 30 cmH2O).**

2. How can the expiratory hold maneuver be used as a diagnostic? **The expiratory hold maneuver provides us with autoPEEP information. An autoPEEP of 0 means there is no autoPEEP occurring. Any positive autoPEEP value means autoPEEP is occurring. To fix this, we need to increase the I:E ratio to reflect a longer E-time. AutoPEEP indicates air trapping, therefore we need to allow longer exhalation times. If you wanted to increase the RR of your mechanically ventilated patient and were concerned it was 'too high' of a RR, you could set the RR and then you could preform the expiratory hold maneuver to check autoPEEP. Therefore, the expiratory hold maneuver can tell us if our RR is safe or if it is too high.**

## PRACTICE SESSION #9:

1. Describe how a transport ventilator is different from a hospital ventilator? **There are multiple examples of the transport ventilator pre- calculating values, such as when you're choosing patient size (adult, pediatric, infant). The tubing diameter is standard and we typically have 2 sizes: adult and pediatric. This creates dead space and pressure issues and without knowing how to clinically navigate around these 'precalcuations' you could get confused with respect to the transport ventilator.**

2. Will applying an ICU ventilator's settings to your transport ventilator without alarms sounding be commonplace? Explain. **No, this will be uncommon. Since there are several 'precalculations' associated with the transport ventilator, it is likely that you'll replicate an ICU ventilators settings on a transport ventilator without alarms. Most likely you'll have to teak your numbers initially to ensure the patient receives what you want them to receive.**

**1.** Describe how to initiate mechanical ventilation on a patient without pulmonary pathophysiology and with normal hemodynamics. **Ensure their blood pressure is acceptable or begin resuscitating them. Determine if they acidotic with a yes to any of these questions 1) low pH, 2) Kussmauls- like RR present, 3) high EtCO2? If they are acidotic, start with a minute ventilation of 9 L/min, and if they are not acidotic start with a minute ventilation between 6-8 L/min. Calculate their IBW and multiply it by the factor for tidal volume (5-8 cc/kg). The result is their ideal tidal volume. Take your chosen minute ventilation and divide it by the ideal tidal volume. This results in the RR. Set the Vt and RR on the ventilator. If you're wanting to use pressure control ventilation, set a PC of 20 and then titration it up or down to achieve a Vte that is close to what you originally calculated the Vt to be. Set FiO2 at 1.0, PEEP between 3-5 cmH2O, and I:E at 1:2 (if the patient is not a pediatric or otherwise have an air trapping pathophysiology).**

2. Your patient is a DKA patient with a pH of 7.3. Describe how to initiate mechanical ventilation on this patient. **These patients will need more minute ventilation to keep up with their acid off load from their respiratory system. NEVER apply a minute ventilation in normal range on these patients. Ensure their blood pressure is acceptable or begin resuscitating them. They are acidotic so being with a minute ventilation of 9 L/min. Calculate their IBW and multiply it by the factor for tidal volume (5-8 cc/kg). The result is their ideal tidal volume. Take your chosen minute ventilation and divide it by the ideal tidal volume. This results in the RR. Set the Vt and RR on the ventilator. If you're wanting to use pressure control ventilation, set a PC of 20 and then titration it up or down to achieve a Vte that is close to what you**

originally calculated the Vt to be. Set FiO2 at 1.0, PEEP between 3-5 cmH2O, and I:E at 1:2 (if the patient is not a pediatric or otherwise have an air trapping pathophysiology).


## PRACTICE SESSION #11:

1. Describe how to initiate mechanical ventilation on a patient exhibiting a closed head injury and increased ICP. **In theory, you may want to aim for a PEEP under 8, but this information is unsubstantiated in the literature. Otherwise, follow the universal approach. Ensure their blood pressure is acceptable or begin resuscitating them. Determine if they acidotic with a yes to any of these questions 1) low pH, 2) Kussmauls-like RR present, 3) high EtCO2? If they are acidotic, start with a minute ventilation of 9 L/min, and if they are not acidotic start with a minute ventilation between 6-8 L/min. Calculate their IBW and multiply it by the factor for tidal volume (5-8 cc/kg). The result is their ideal tidal volume. Take your chosen minute ventilation and divide it by the ideal tidal volume. This results in the RR. Set the Vt and RR on the ventilator. If you're wanting to use pressure control ventilation, set a PC of 20 and then titration it up or down to achieve a Vte that is close to what you originally calculated the Vt to be. Set FiO2 at 1.0, PEEP between 3-5 cmH2O (consider keeping < 8 cmH2O), and I:E at 1:2 (if the patient is not a pediatric or otherwise have an air trapping pathophysiology).**

2. Your patient is an asthmatic and has been self-medicating for 24 hours and now requires intubation. Describe how to initiate mechanical ventilation on this patient. We know that this patient will need longer E-times to combat the air trapping nature of asthma. **Ensure their blood pressure**

is acceptable or begin resuscitating them. Determine if they acidotic with a yes to any of these questions 1) low pH, 2) Kussmauls- like RR present, 3) high EtCO2? If they are acidotic, start with a minute ventilation of 9 L/min, and if they are not acidotic start with a minute ventilation between 6-8 L/min. Calculate their IBW and multiply it by the factor for tidal volume (5-8 cc/kg). The result is their ideal tidal volume. Take your chosen minute ventilation and divide it by the ideal tidal volume. This results in the RR. Set the Vt and RR on the ventilator. If you're wanting to use pressure control ventilation, set a PC of 20 and then titration it up or down to achieve a Vte that is close to what you originally calculated the Vt to be. Set FiO2 at 1.0, PEEP between 3-5 cmH2O, and I:E at 1:5 or 1:6.

## PRACTICE SESSION #12:

1.  Describe how to initiate mechanical ventilation on a patient low blood pressure. **We first need to aggressively attack the blood pressure. Fluids, blood products (for trauma patients requiring blood replacement), and pressors as needed (never first line in trauma). Also, you. Could consider a hypotension strategy: higher pressures and less RR, but still targeting a particular minute ventilation. Perhaps administer 1 L or NS or LR fluid bonus. Determine if they acidotic with a yes to any of these questions 1) low pH, 2) Kussmauls-like RR present, 3) high EtCO2? If they are acidotic, start with a minute ventilation of 9 L/min, and if they are not acidotic start with a minute ventilation between 6-8 L/min. Calculate their IBW and multiply it by the factor for tidal volume (5-8 cc/kg). The result is their ideal tidal volume. Take your chosen minute ventilation and divide it by the ideal tidal volume. This results in the RR. Set the Vt and RR on the ventilator. If you're wanting to use pressure control ventilation, set a PC of 20 and then titration it up or**

down to achieve a Vte that is close to what you originally calculated the Vt to be. Set FiO2 at 1.0, PEEP between 3-5 cmH2O, and I:E at 1:2 (if the patient is not a pediatric or otherwise have an air trapping pathophysiology).

2. Your patient is an ARDS patient. Describe how to initiate mechanical ventilation on this patient. **It would most likely be wise to begin on pressure control ventilation. If you decide to go with volume ventilation, be diligent in monitoring the plateau pressures. Ensure their blood pressure is acceptable or begin resuscitating them. Determine if they acidotic with a yes to any of these questions 1) low pH, 2) Kussmauls-like RR present, 3) high EtCO2? If they are acidotic, start with a minute ventilation of 9 L/min, and if they are not acidotic start with a minute ventilation between 6-8 L/min. Calculate their IBW and multiply it by the factor for tidal volume (5-8 cc/kg). The result is their ideal tidal volume. Take your chosen minute ventilation and divide it by the ideal tidal volume. This results in the RR. Set the Vt and RR on the ventilator. If you're wanting to use pressure control ventilation, set a PC of 20 and then titration it up or down to achieve a Vte that is close to what you originally calculated the Vt to be. Set FiO2 at 1.0, PEEP between 3-5 cmH2O, and I:E at 1:2 (if the patient is not a pediatric or otherwise have an air trapping pathophysiology).**

PRACTICE SESSION #13:

1. Explain why perfusion is important to the mechanically ventilated patient. **Without perfusion, most specifically a present distal pulse, then we will not be to be able to trust our governing vital signs: SpO2 and EtCO2.**

2. How can low perfusion and blood pressure affect the EtCO2 and SpO2. **If we do not have a distal pulse, then**

we are most likely not perfusing our tissues, thus SpO2 will be low and the EtCO2 will become low as well. After perfusion is re-established, then the SpO2 should rise and the EtCO2 will spike to over normal levels.

## PRACTICE SESSION #14:

1. Your patient is a 9 year old trauma patient. What is the typical minute ventilation of a patient this age. **This patient's normal minute ventilation is most likely 2-4 L/min. Adults have a normal minute ventilation of 4-8 L/min, pediatric's normal ventilation is 2-4 L/min, and infants is between 0.5-2 L/min.**

2. List the 3 questions needed to identify if a patient is acidotic. **To determine if they acidotic, ask the following questions. If they answer with a yes to any of these questions 1) low pH, 2) Kussmauls- like RR present, 3) high EtCO2?**

## PRACTICE SESSION #15:

1. Calculate the IBW, ITV, and RR of a patient who is 6'4", male, and who needs a VE of 11 L/min. **The IBW is 86.8 (2.3 x 16 + 50). The ITV range would be 434-693 cc (5-8 cc/kg x 86.8 kg). The RR will need to be 25/min with an ITV of 434cc, and would need to be 15/min with an ITV of 693 cc.**

2. Calculate the IBW, ITV, and RR of a patient who is 5'7", female, and who needs a VE of 7 L/min. **The IBW is 61.6 (2.3 x 7 + 45.5). The ITV range would be 308-493 cc (5-8 cc/kg x 61.6 kg). The RR will need to be 23/min with an ITV of 308 cc, and would need to be 14/min with an ITV of 493 cc.**

3. Calculate the IBW, ITV, and RR of a patient who is 6'1", male,

and who needs a VE of 8 L/min. **The IBW is 79.9 (2.3 x 13 + 50). The ITV range would be 400-639 cc (5-8 cc/kg x 79.9 kg). The RR will need to be 20/min with an ITV of 400 cc, and would need to be 13/min with an ITV of 639 cc.**

## PRACTICE SESSION #16:

1. Determine the I;E ratio, FiO2, and PEEP on the following patient: 4 month old with pneumonia. **This patient most likely would benefit from oxygen, so begin the FiO2 at 1.0 and titration down as quickly as possible to prevent hyperopia. Additionally, begin PEEP at 5 cmH2O to assist with oxygenation. The I:E ratio needs to reflect a longer E-time, so perhaps begin at 1:5. Later, you could assess the expiratory hold maneuver to evaluate for autoPEEP.**

2. Determine the I:E ratio, FiO2, and PEEP on the following patient: 35 y/o trauma patient with hypoxia and hypotension. **Hopefully, you would begin working on the blood pressure early. This patient most likely would benefit from oxygen, so begin the FiO2 at 1.0 and titrate down as quickly as possible to prevent hyperopia. Additionally, begin PEEP at 5 cmH2O to assist with oxygenation. The I:E ratio needs to be initiated at 1:2 because there is no evidence to support an I:E ratio with a longer E-time.**

3. Determine the I;E ratio, FiO2, and PEEP on the following patient: 21 y/o exhibiting shortness of breath and wheezes. **Just like the first patient, this patient has an air trapping pathophysiology and will most likely need longer E-times. This patient most likely would benefit from oxygen, so begin the FiO2 at 1.0 and titration down as quickly as possible to prevent hyperopia. Additionally, begin PEEP at 5 cmH2O to assist with oxygenation. The I:E ratio needs to reflect a longer E-time, so perhaps begin at 1:5. Later, you could assess the expiratory hold maneuver to evaluate for autoPEEP.**

## PRACTICE SESSION #17:

1. Your expected VE is 6 L/min and the ventilator is displaying a VE of 3 L/min. What should you investigate next? **Next you should investigate the two possibilities that would cause a lower minute ventilation than what was set: RR and Vt. First, look to the set RR and ensure it matches the f, or the actual number of times the patient's chest rises and falls. If that matched, then I would then investigate the Vte to see if it matched the set Vt.**

2. You are troubleshooting a high minute ventilation alarm and note a RR of 16, VE of 9 L/min, and f of 22. What needs to be done to correct the high minute ventilation alarm? **In this particular case it is quite easy to identify the problem. The RR is set to 16/min but the frequency is observed at 22/min. Therefore, it makes complete sense that the minute ventilation alarm would go off. Sedate this patient, or turn up the sensitivity setting.**

3. You have set the ventilator to deliver a Vt of 550 and it only delivers 501. Does this represent a significant dead space problem? **No, not in this case. If the Vte is within +/- 50 cmH2O of the set Vt, then it can be considered close enough. When there is a difference between Vte and Vt within 50 cmH2O, it is easy to fix, typically by simply adding a single breath per minute of RR.**

## PRACTICE SESSION #18:

1. A high pressure alarm sounds and you not a PIP of 57 and a pPlat of 48? What is the significance of these findings? **A high PIP and a high pPlat indicates a compliance problem. The patient should immediately be changed to pressure control ventilation.**

2. The monitored data on the ventilator reads PIP 32 and pPlat of 29. What is the significance of these findings? **These are both normal findings.**

3. A high pressure alarm sounds and you not a PIP of 54 and a pPlat of 22? What is the significance of these findings? **A high PIP and normal pPlat indicates an airway resistance problem. A review of the DOPE acronym could quickly reveal the answer.**

## PRACTICE SESSION #19:

1. Your patient has the following ventilator findings: RR 16, Vt 575, I:E 1:2, VE 9.1, SpO2 92, EtCO2 48, Pplat 17, Vte 572, and AutoPEEP 0. What changes to the ventilator can be made to correct the abnormal values? **The SpO2 is low and can be increased by either adding more FiO2 or PEEP. The EtCO2 is also elevated, and that can be fixed by increasing RR, Vt, or PC.**

2. Your patient has the following ventilator findings: RR vent assisted at 16 or 18, SpO2 98%, EtCO2 is 51, VE 8.9, f 18, Vte 556, PIP 17, Pplat 13, and AutoPEEP 0. What changes to the ventilator can be made to correct the abnormal values? **In this case, the SpO2 is perfect, but the EtCO2 is high, and that can be fixed by increasing RR, Vt, or PC.**

## PRACTICE SESSION #20:

1. You patient has an EtCO2 of 28 mmHg and a pH of 7.24. Why would reducing minute ventilation in this case be dangerous. **If you remember nothing else about caveats in changing minute ventilation to effect a change in EtCO2, be sure to remember that a low pH and a low EtCO2 is dangerous. This is the profile of metabolic acidosis. When pH is low, the higher pCO2 (or EtCO2) becomes. As pCO2 (or EtCO2) gets larger, it will drop pH further. Therefore, if you arrive and apply a ventilator to a metabolic acidosis patient and begin dropping minute ventilation (thus increasing pCO2), you essentially are further dropping pH.**

2. Using Winter's formula, calculate the corrected pCO2 from the following data: pH 7.25, pCO2 30, HCO3 12, pO2 99, BE -1. **Winter's formula is PCO2 = 1.5 x (HCO3) + 8 +/- 2, so in this case the corrected PCO2 is 1.5 x 12 + 8 = 26 +/- 2, or 24-28 mmHg. This is incredibly low. The pH is also low, so this is the case where you titrate minute ventilation to target a EtCO2 between 24-28 mmHg. This will prevent the pH from falling further.**

## PRACTICE SESSION #21:

1. Why is it important to unclamp the endotracheal tube when your transport ventilator is attempting to deliver positive breaths? **The entire purpose of clamping the endotracheal tube is executed to maintain the gaseous splinting of the airway. This splinting is essentially holding open the airway and is preventing atelectasis. Once sick and inflamed alveoli collapse, it takes hours to re-recruit all the alveoli again. Therefore, to keep alveolis open, the endotracheal tube is unclamped the moment the transport ventilator is trying to advance air into the patient's lungs. This way no recruitment, or splinting, is lost.**

2. You are about to clamp a patient's endotracheal tube for the first time and want to be prepared for any complications. What are some complications that can occur with this procedure? **The biggest fear, and a significant complication, is inadvertently cutting the endotracheal tube during clamping. This is why it is imperative that you use a gauze around the endotracheal tube durning clamping. The is the primary complication to worry about with this procedure.**

## PRACTICE SESSION #22:

1. You have a patient with CHF and you decide to attempt non-invasive positive pressure ventilation. Currently, the patient has these findings: HR 102, RR 24, SpO2 85, and EtCO2 41. Which type of NPPV is warranted here? **There is only an oxygenation problem here, therefore, CPAP is the appropriate NPPV mode.**

2. Your COPD patient is short of breath and has the following findings: HR 82, RR 18, SpO2 88, and EtCO2 61. Which type of NPPV is warranted here? **This particular case has both an oxygenation and a ventilation problem, therefore, could benefit from BPAP.**

## PRACTICE SESSION #23:

1. You have an oxygen tank that is 660 L in capacity and has a max fill pressure of 1900 PSI. What is the cal factor for this oxygen tank? **Cal factor for an oxygen tank is capacity in L divided by the max fill pressure. In this case, 660/1900 = 0.347, therefore, the cal factor is 0.347 for this tank.**

2. Your ventilated patient has a minute ventilation of 6 L/min and an FiO2 of 0.7. What is this patient's ventilator liter flow? **Liter flow for a ventilator is minute ventilation (Vte x f) multiplied by the FiO2. In this case, the minute ventilation is provided as well as the FiO2 making the calculation very easy. The ventilator liter flow in this case is 6 L/min x 0.7 FiO2 = 4.2 L/min.**

3. You have an oxygen tank that is 500 L in capacity and has a max fill pressure of 2100 PSI. Your ventilated patient has a minute ventilation of 9 L/min and an FiO2 of 0.9. Your oxygen tank is currently at 1600 PSI. What is the duration of your oxygen tank? **Oxygen tank cal factor is 500/2100 = 0.238. Oxygen duration for this tank is (0.238 x 1600 PSI)/8.1 (vent liter flow) = 47 minutes of duration.**

## PRACTICE SESSION #24:

1. You have set an I:E ratio for your patient who is having an asthmatic attack. How can you identify if this I:E ratio is appropriate? **Execute an expiratory hold maneuver; this provides you with the autoPEEP value. Continue to choose longer E-times until the autoPEEP is zero. Ultimately, make I:E ratio changes (in favor of longer E-times) until autoPEEP goes away. If on your first measurement autoPEEP is observed at zero, then there is no breath stacking occurring.**

2. Explain how we can change our treatment by utilizing the inspiratory hold maneuver. **The inspiratory hold maneuver provides us with plateau pressure. If we had our patient on volume on troll ventilation, they experienced high airway pressures, and discovered a high plateau pressures, we could then change our treatment from volume control ventilation to pressure control ventilation and protect the patient's lungs.**

## PRACTICE SESSION #25:

1. Your patient is in ARDS and you have had to titrate up PEEP to 17 cmH2O to be able to oxygenate the patient. You notice a low minute ventilation alarm sounding. Explain why this alarm sounded. **As you raise PEEP, you take away Vte. BE PREPARED FOR THIS. If you see a lower Vte or VE, or if you see a trending upward EtCO2, do what you are trained to do- increase either RR, Vt, or PC to increase the minute ventilation.**

2. You change the RR on your patient and later notice that they are autoPEEPing. Explain why this happened. **The faster you set the RR, the less time you have to exhale, therefore, you are risking breath stacking. So, if you increase the RR and then run a exipratory hold maneuver**

out of good measure and identify autoPEEPing is occurring, then you'll need to increase the I:E ratio in favor of longer E-times to allow for trapped gases to escape.

# ABOUT THE AUTHOR

Charlie Swearingen first conceived the dream of becoming a flight clinician while he was still in paramedic school. He decided that instead of blithely waiting for a position to become available, he would begin arming himself with the professional achievements that would eventually earn him a spot on a revered, level 1 helicopter in Mississippi. He is in the middle of a PhD in physiology, is an educator for the world's largest air medical service provider, and also is a world class athlete on the US National Men's Sitting volleyball team. Years after his inaugural medical flight, he decided to focus his learning efforts on the mechanical ventilator. His ultimate goal is to improve the quality of care delivered to his patients. By advancing the knowledge of transport ventilator management, he is confident that this goal can be achieved.